THE
HEALER'S
PROCESS

"Katherine writes about the mystical and unexplainable in such a grounded, clear way that you accept your magic as just a natural way of being. When you have this and realize it, you get to really live your purpose! This incredible book is destined to be a staple on every healer's shelf."

EBONIE ALLARD
adhd Mystic, Artist, and Author of *Misfit to Maven*

"There are plenty of people who 'talk a good talk.' And then there is Katherine. Everything she does, everything she creates, emanates her boundless commitment to self-honoring, spiritual seeing, profound healing, and authentic self-expression. There are few places that Katherine is unwilling to go, which makes her a rare and precious guide."

ROSY ARONSON, PH.D.,
Author of *Walking a Fine Line: Becoming a Professional Wisdom Keeper in the Healing Arts*

"*The Healers Process* is a strategic surrender to what's possible for all healers. The book provides the structure and valuable tools to cultivate deeper healing abilities while honoring the beauty that unfolds as we come back to wholeness."

ODYSSEUS ANDRIANOS
Author of *Shadow Awakening*

"The world needs more people willing to step into the sacred role of healer. Katherine holds your hand through these pages so that you can move past the blocks, fears, and challenges and bring your unique and powerful magic to the world."

MAURA RASSMAN-GWIAZDA
Creator Aerial Somatic Therapy, Author of *Forever Blue*

"I've known Katherine Bird for nearly a decade and have been so consistently impressed with her dedication to the process of spiritual illumination and healing. Katherine has a powerful and natural way of holding open the mystical door of possibility with genuine care and ethics we should all strive for as transformational leaders."

MATT KREINHEDER
Author of *Awakening The Mystics*

"In *The Healer's Process*, Katherine stands as a luminous guide for those ready to fully embrace their magic with unshakeable integrity and ethics. Her work not only illuminates the path to authentic healing and service but also invites you into a deeper communion with your innate powers. A must-read for any healer seeking to transform their practice and the world."

DESTIN GERIK
Men's Coach, Author of *The Evolved Masculine*

"There is no question that *The Healer's Process* work gave me the confidence to step into my power as a creator and facilitator. Katherine's work supports those called to a life of aligned and ethical service. Anyone who is considering going into healing and spiritual facilitation work should do themselves a favor and make sure this book is on their shelf."

ARDEN LEIGH
creator of The Re-Patterning Project

"Katherine is not only a master healer, but also a masterful teacher. This book translates esoteric concepts of healership and energy medicine into tangible, practical tools and techniques that support new, budding intuitive healers and well-established, seasoned practitioners alike. *The Healer's Process* belongs on every healer's reading list."

MICHELLE HAWK
Shaman, Alchemist, Spiritual Mentor

"I studied *The Healer's Process* with Katherine when I noticed I tended to take on the energies of my coaching clients. I wanted to learn practical tools to ensure I brought my best service forward while caring for myself. In the process, I had new gifts come online that have really shifted the way I do my work. I'm so grateful Kat has decided to make this deep and practical work accessible in this book! Thank you!"

DARLA LEDOUX
Founder of Sourced and Author of *Shift the Field*

THE HEALER'S PROCESS

INNER WORK & SKILL DEVELOPMENT
TO FULFILL YOUR SACRED PURPOSE

KATHERINE **BIRD**

ILLUSTRATIONS BY JANELLE DESPOT

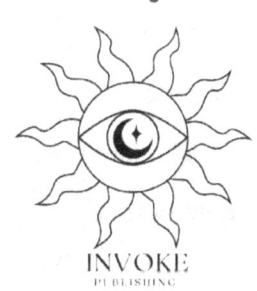

INVOKE
PUBLISHING

For rights and permissions, please contact:

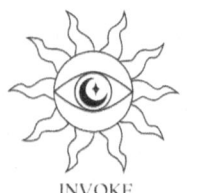

Invoke Publishing

www.invokepublishing.com

Santa Fe, New Mexico

INVOKE
PUBLISHING

DEDICATION

This book is dedicated to my many teachers. I have been blessed to study and train with true masters. I honor all those who held me on my path and gave me the tools to transform my life and work.

I firmly acknowledge Mayaya, my first spiritual and energetic teacher. As she loves to tell the story, I was a bud tightly held when first we met.

I am grateful for my dear friends, loves, and collaborators who have encouraged and inspired me, especially Michelle, Taylore, Charmaine, and Will, who seem to have always been.

I thank my clients and students for trusting me and walking with me side by side on this incredible path of healing.

Thank you, Earth Mother, for holding and teaching me each day.

I acknowledge my ancestors, spirit guides and teachers, the ancient ones, and healers who sing through me. I know that I am truly blessed.

For my parents, who encouraged my wildness and expression.

Thank you, thank you, thank you, thank you.

CONTENTS

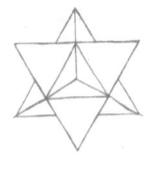

MY CALLING

I call all those ready to step into mastery, to hold their medicine, to fulfill their sacred work.

I call all those who are part of the transformation of consciousness, those here to serve, to hold space for healing, and those committed to healing themselves.

I call those ready to move past the blocks, thoughts, beliefs, and wounds from this lifetime or any other.

I call those ready to train, to master, to understand, to receive the tools they most need to authentically express.

I call the healers, the shamans, the channels, the guides, all those committed to be, the beingness that they are, to stand as transformational beacons of light on this planet so that others may, in contact with them, also transform.

I call those committed. I call those in need.

I call those ready. I call those.

ABOUT THE AUTHOR

I did not expect my life to lead me to these pages. I never intended to be a healer or a spiritual guide. These were not options given out on career day. They were not words written on a paper kite and taped to the wall in elementary school.

Life has intelligence beyond me and has offered me a glimpse into worlds many see as fiction or fanciful thinking.

Blasted open. Shot through with power and shifted in an instant. This could describe my initial awakening. I was thrust into deep channel states, energetic activations, hours upon hours of visions, messages, and transmissions. The shift in vibration that occurred for me was intense—at times, both frightening and filled with wonder. Able to do little else but process this new reality, I sunk into studying my energy system—healing my physical and emotional bodies and learning the tools I needed to bring my new being into the world.

I trained with masters in anatomy and physiology, movement and sacred dance, alchemy, yoga, medical qi gong, shamanism, meditation, channeling, structural to-the-bone body-work, energy practices, herbalism and nutrition, reiki, tantra, and other modalities. Later I sought mentors to help me understand the nuts and bolts of making a living through my authentic expression. I have integrated these with my inner remembrances and explorations to offer healing and guidance for those ready to evolve.

Early on, I heard the message, "You are a healer." This seemed impossible as I felt broken in many ways, but I chose to listen and follow the little inner voice, spurring me forward. My awakening was not easy and may have seemed a type of madness. I had to fight through blocks that kept me from being actualized. I had to stabilize, ground, cultivate, and heal. This created a powerful portal that propelled me toward my destiny. I was offered a way to wake up, join my collaborators in the unseen and seen worlds, and do the work I came here to do.

In this process, I met past lives, pulling through their wisdom. I've unpacked societal conditionings that taught me to remain small and not express what I see, hear, or know. I've sat with my wounds, transforming trauma into light. I've held and danced with my inner child, met my parts, called my soul fragments home, and learned the lesson of surrender over and over again. I've formed deep relationships with my guides and the natural world. I am grateful that this journey has allowed me to remember myself.

My path, so clearly laid out before me, is one of being a bridge for others. People come to me to awaken their energy and potential. They bring their fears and shame. They wonder about their sanity and place in the world. They come to me when they realize they have the potential to be great healers, leaders, channels, and mystics, even if they haven't fully embraced it yet. My arduous journey of awakening informs my unwavering support for those navigating this complex experience.

In my professional career, I have supported people through hands-on and distance physical, energetic, and shamanic healing, practice cultivation, and transformational retreats and events. I am blessed to have incredible collaborators, facilitating men's work with Charmaine Haworth, hosting shamanism, alchemy, other retreats and trainings, and a podcast, "Shaman Sister Sessions," with Michelle Hawk. I mentor healers, channels, shamans, therapists, medicine people, coaches, executives, and entrepreneurs. I regularly teach healing, channeling, energy practices, and Qi Gong in my courses, including "5 Elements Alchemy," "Open Your Channel," and "The Healer's Process" (where I lead you through the work in this book) and other workshops and online courses.

I constantly push myself to learn, experience more, and confront shadows that keep me held back, and I do the same for those who come to me for help. In alignment with striving to be a better practitioner and person, I study internal alchemy and Daoist mysticism, Buddhist philosophy, psychology, meditation, and somatic and energy practices.

The Healer's Process is an important part of my mission because I needed this support along my path. I didn't understand my gifts or how to translate them into helping others. I was scared of what was coming through me. I was afraid of being seen. I underwent a long healing process and intense training with my mentors and guides.

Long ago, I was told that I would help others. That we would come together to be a beacon of light. That I was to lead, share, and be seen. This is what I have placed inside these pages. My beacon of light. So that you may shine brighter and bring your work to the world faster.

I work with people in group programs and one on one. For more on my work, head over to my website or social media:

katherinebird.com

facebook.com/KatherineBird711/

instagram.com/katherinebird711/

YouTube: @KatherineBird; @ShamanSisterSessions - podcast

Special Book Bonus Resources: Gain access to free special resources and education associated with The Healer's Process: https://katherinebird.com/the-healers-process-bonus/

PROLOGUE

People allow me into their hearts, minds, and energy systems; they reveal themselves to me. Why? Why do they trust me? Because with the fullness of my heart and all that I am, I trust myself to hold space for them—no matter what comes up. I trust my training and what has emerged from years of dedication to my craft. I trust my spirit guides, mentors, and healers that I work with from the unseen realms. The relationships I have with them are reciprocal and evolving. I trust them to guide my words and hands. I am consistent in my devotion, offerings, and recognition of their support in every aspect of my life. I trust my collaborators and colleagues to support me and call me out if I am out of alignment or integrity. I trust the community I train to take what I am offering and use it to benefit the Earth and her people, animals, and ecosystems. I trust my path to rise to meet me and that every interaction I have is an opportunity for growth and healing.

This hasn't always been the case. I've experienced doubt and fear and attempted to conceal my true self. I've spent many years integrating my gifts and their surrounding shadows. It's been a long road to discovering my unique, authentic voice as a healer and guide. Along the way, I've made mistakes. I've sometimes become overwhelmed, confused, and caught up in my ego. There are lessons I've learned the hard way. My way through these challenges has been to maintain a focused devotion to energy, spirit, ethics, practices, and self-inquiry.

At one time, I wondered why I received so many messages about teaching or explaining concepts while doing them. I know now. I am a teacher, and my greatest gift to offer is empowering and supporting healers and magic people. The difficulty of my path required me to develop a level of mastery that is ultimately intended for the service of others.

We are in a time of collective shift. Transformations are rarely easy. Many have come here with valuable abilities and awareness to support the underlying current of change occurring on the planet. I am committed, as perhaps you are, to helping bring about a collective shift in consciousness and to support the healing of all people as we reconnect to our intrinsic natures. This is fundamental to shifting the current environmental and social challenges that contribute to suffering and the destruction of life on Earth. We will change the world. One person healed of their deep wounds reverberates out to touch all. The purpose of this book is to support you to support awakening humanity—all hands on deck.

How will you show up for this powerful moment?

How do you know what type of healer you are and how you work?

How do you become a fully actualized, authentic, and effective healer?

How can you achieve your mission of activating and supporting all those you come in contact with?

The Healer's Process will help answer these questions. When you study and follow this process, you will find you are sourced, grounded, and available. Magic is given space to enter, healing shows itself, and the truth emerges from the shadows.

WELCOME TO THE HEALER'S PROCESS

Master healers master themselves.

Great healers study many disciplines and crafts, born on the backs of profound lineages. You, too, are on this journey of discovery. If you are called to be a healer, it is already in your bones and blood.

You might not resonate with the title of healer. You may never do sessions with individual people. You may be called to community or Earth healing. You may be called to heal yourself and your lineages, which is also a great service to the world.

The Healer's Process gives you the tools and practices to work on yourself, move through your healing and awakening, ground in your energetic and spiritual practices, and establish the landscape for your evolved expression in the world. You will be guided to work personally through your process and discover how to translate the teachings into your unique modalities and ways of being a healing presence.

This book is a powerful combination of healing modalities and discoveries called "The Healer's Process."™ This is about your journey of discovering your innate healing and spiritual abilities while tracking simple, repeatable steps that every healing session contains. You can use this book entirely in service to your own growth or allow it to catalyze your healing work for others. If you do any healing, spiritual, or ceremonial work, the lessons here will directly translate, enhancing your capacity and experiences. This book can be used with my course or as a standalone guide.

The companion *Healer's Process Practice Manual* contains energy practices and step-by-step guidance for deepening into The Healer's Process concepts. Incorporating the practices will help you get the most out of the teachings. Along with the practices, you will find further clarifications and teachings. In the book's text, you will find references to the companion practices in [brackets] so you can switch between the texts. This text is a complete guide, even if you do not have the practice manual.

The Healer's Process seeks to empower you by honoring your intuitive gifts and inner knowing with a process that will guide you and your client more effectively—allowing you to do more fulfilling work. The Process will enable you to build more power, presence, and confidence in your work and life.

I am glad you are on this journey with me.

WHAT IS A HEALER?

A healer is a space in which healing happens.

The term "healer" is loaded. Many debate its meaning, and some argue that an individual can't heal another. This is basically true. Healing is co-creation with the Divine, the individual, connections to helpful energies, and the Universal life force that runs through all. We are all healers. Our bodies and spirits are remarkable healing entities all on their own. These healing abilities are constantly at work within us.

Some say "healer" and "healing" imply someone is broken and needs fixing, but we are already whole and only need to realize it. In essence, this is also true. However, there is a journey that individuals go through to come to this profound realization, which I believe is one of the purposes of our existence on Earth. If you have a significant illness, are in deep debt, or are in an abusive relationship, you can't just say, "I am fine, I am whole, I am healed," and everything goes away. The journey must be taken. Aspects must be explored, felt, expressed, shifted, and integrated.

Saying, "You are already whole," can evoke shame when one feels an issue needs attention or support. This true but confusing statement can be used to mean that affirming wholeness alone will protect you from being uncomfortable. Affirmations and visualizations are incredible tools, but so are somatic therapy, energy work, soul work, and many other therapeutic processes.

Some also take the spiritual truth that nothing is broken or needs fixing to mean, "I am as I am, and that is perfect." This can lead to avoiding shadow work and confronting fears. Some feel that going into their challenging aspects proves they have been omitted from the wholeness club everyone else enjoys. These beliefs can stop self-inquiry and striving to escape pain instead of being with it, avoiding parts of self that are seen as not of the light and not of wholeness. Wholeness is a fully integrated self, the light, and the shadow, falling in love with all aspects. A healer is a space in which this integration can take place.

I use the term "healer" to mean anyone who brings healing to the world and "healing" to mean a process of returning to the whole.

The Work of a Healer

Healing is an empowering journey, and you, the guide, hold that your client is already aware of their wholeness. It has already happened, is already done, but you're not afraid of going into anything that comes up in the process of unfolding toward that truth. You draw attention to what needs noticing. You call in supportive energies. You give people permission to travel into painful places they would otherwise not dare to tread. You help remove blockages, which impede the system's natural ability to heal. Due to your training, experience, and innate gifts, you inspire trust so that others may find their way home to themselves. Healers walk in many forms. You might be drawn to hands-on healing, subtle energy work, counseling or coaching, Western or Eastern medical modalities, plant medicine, shamanic works, or any other way that space is created with the intention of healing.

Some people receive instant, profound healing. Others must address other aspects of their lives, including anything (from food to relationships to careers), to work through their healing and become empowered through their experiences. If you can integrate their soul parts back into their body, clear stagnancies, bring in beneficial energies, and give them access to the wisdom of their highest self and tools for care at home, they will naturally heal themselves.

The Healer's Process is divided into six chapters, each with practical exercises and journaling prompts for self-exploration, and I will encourage you, again and again, to look and feel deeply when certain words or phrases trigger emotions within you. If you feel very called to the work and title of healer, this is something to look at and consider. It also holds information if you are repulsed by it or don't want to take on the label. We will explore more in the section on "healer archetypes." Throughout the text, I offer ways to challenge your conception of who you are and what your role is as a healer. I will use other challenging words, such as shaman (there is much more to be said about this title in The Sacred Container section). I invite you to keep an open mind and explore your depths when you encounter concepts and words that make you uncomfortable. Through the Healer's Process and your work, you will have a much clearer understanding and connection to the healer that you are.

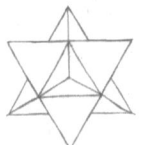

SENSITIVE SOUL

You, of the sensitive soul, know you are needed.

You have worn empathy as a wound, yet it is your sword.

You are here to feel.

Awaken us to our intuitive animal natures.

Express the beauty of our connection to the Divine.

Please don't hide.

Don't shrink away from uncomfortable places.

Don't be afraid that we will see your tears.

For your tears are jewels refracting the depths of your being.

You of the sensitive soul.

Your time is now.

You are called to hold space for all of our transformations.

Tell us what you feel, what you know, what is right and in alignment.

Hold your ground.

Learn protection.

But, be ready to open fully to pull through the healing we need.

You of the sensitive soul,

Please . . .

Please . . .

Know you are needed.

HEAL YOURSELF TO
KNOW HEALING

Healing work transmits the frequency of who you are.
Thus, all healing work is a refinement of self.

T his soul path calls out from beyond, teases us into its web, and often arises through the deep journey of healing personal pain, illness, or trauma. Healing ourselves is a vital part of the journey, and initiation often arises through self-healing, which pushes us into a life of service. Inner work and self-refinement are necessary. We are drawn to magical gifts, abilities, and skills, but deep personal healing must accompany the path so the work offered remains beneficial at every stage of development.

When I was twenty, I was an actor and a stuntperson. Bad falls and being dropped on my head resulted in a spine twisted and compressed. I lived in constant pain for years. Healing my physical body led me to seek talented healers, encompassing many modalities as I mastered self-care practices. I studied anatomy, kinesiology, massage, and structural bodywork. I healed myself and, in the process, became highly compassionate to all those who live with pain as I had known it so well. I became an advocate of self-care and somatic experiencing.

Further series of initiations were born from a radical energetic and spiritual awakening after going off psychotropic medications, which I'd been taking since I was fifteen. This awakening blasted through my system and created havoc. I began channeling, moving extreme amounts of energy, having visions, feeling everything intensely, and healing deep wounds from many lifetimes. I sought out healers and masters of energy, movement, and spiritual practice to help me navigate my newfound gifts and experiences. The process required deep inner work, energetic and spiritual skill development, trauma release, rebalancing my nervous system, and bringing many years of repressed emotions into the light.

I received the message that I was a healer but had to heal myself to understand how to walk this path.

The next stage was coming out as a healer, refining my gifts, and determining how to bring them to the world. I have devoted myself to this act of service, which is my deepest soul's code. Along the way, I have felt lost, alone, scared, overwhelmed, and confused. Yet, the more I committed to the path, the more it rose to meet me, and the people and practices I needed found me.

Throughout the unfolding years, I have been guided as to the importance of excavating the inner world. Unexamined wounds, beliefs, and motivations will impact us as we achieve power, success, and influence. Radical self-honesty is required, and greed, envy, rage, desire, and aversion can poison a practitioner on the path, becoming a minister of harm instead of healing. We are all human, capable of deviating from our light, and must be willing to do the self-work required to hold this position with ethical integrity.

I want you to know that you are not alone; you have access to the tools to help you navigate the healer's journey: healing yourself, refining your gifts, and bringing them to the world. Like many things, this isn't a linear path but often spirals in on itself as it goes through more profound levels of initiation and healing as you continuously grow into more significant roles of service and mastery.

Finding Your Way

All too often, healers play small. Perhaps you have been deeply drawn to be a healer, but your conditioning doesn't hold space for that possibility. Maybe you've taken the path of massage therapist, yoga teacher, reiki practitioner, or medical professional—but know you are hiding behind modalities and not fully exploring your innate gifts. You may love your bodywork, coaching, or counseling practice, but know there is something more to learn and lean into. *The Healer's Process* empowers you to connect even more deeply to your path as a healer, no matter your expression. The tools and techniques can be integrated into any modality and will inspire you to explore not only what you have learned but also what you are remembering.

In this book, you'll find phrases that I regularly use in my practice. I encourage you to try these out, use what works, throw out what doesn't, modify, play, and allow yourself to be in the moment. Authentic participation is the key to being a powerful healer. My way can be a guiding light, but it isn't "the way." Your approach is what is essential. Like any teacher or guide, I am a light along the path. The path is yours.

You will also find different lineages merging on these pages. This is because I have had the blessing of many teachers. I have studied Eastern, Western, and American systems. I offer you overlaps as best I can as I share energetic anatomy from the perspective of the Daoist (Taoist) lineage and simple relations to Yogic systems such as chakras because you might be familiar with those terms. Working with spirits moves across cultures, and my work has been informed by Spiritism, Indigenous perspectives, my guides, and experience. I intend that the right words meet you to inspire your exploration.

You have been here many times. You have been a healer many times. You know what is right for you. It takes a willingness to be present with your truth. Realization of your truth takes time and attention to nurture forward. You may have shut down your magic, abilities, and awareness for most of your life. This exploration process will give you access to your deep inner knowing—which the world has been waiting for.

The Healer's Process

There is a straightforward formula for creating a healing space and going into your work, either in individual healing sessions or group work. It is also the process of going into practice space for your own healing and personal evolution and comprises the six chapters of The Healer's Process; they are:

1. **I AM**: Uncover your authentic essence, move past blocks and fear, and cultivate your personal power.

2. **Building the Field**: Understand, develop, and work with your energy bodies, build presence, boundaries, and resiliency, heal deep wounds, and be sourced and grounded.

3. **Cleansing and Purification**: Learn tools and techniques to effectively work on yourself and others and protect your space. Discover discernment and clarity in your work.

4. **Sacred Container**: Learn protocols and explore your way of holding a space for healing, as well as how to work with guides and other spiritual and energetic forces.

5. **The Work**: Explore your unique gifts, channeling, and mediumship, how to hold an effective session, and dive into deeper self-work.

6. **Integration**: Learn how to support yourself and others in the healing process, integrate deep and powerful work, and be your best mentor and healer.

View these chapters or sections of the process as points on a spiral. See yourself moving through it—either going from one to the other, back and forth, or moving into the section most called for in every moment. For example, you might shift back to "Cleansing and Purification" after "The Work" to clean up energetic debris and ensure you and your space haven't collected negative energy from the session.

This process provides flexibility and confidence by offering clear guidance on what is required at every moment. Sometimes, shamanic and intuitive practitioners can become so engrossed in "The Work" that they overlook important factors such as grounding, cleansing and purification, setting up and maintaining the sacred container, and other aspects of healing work that will be illuminated throughout the text. This can affect their clients, who may miss out on essential components that make the work more comfortable and effective.

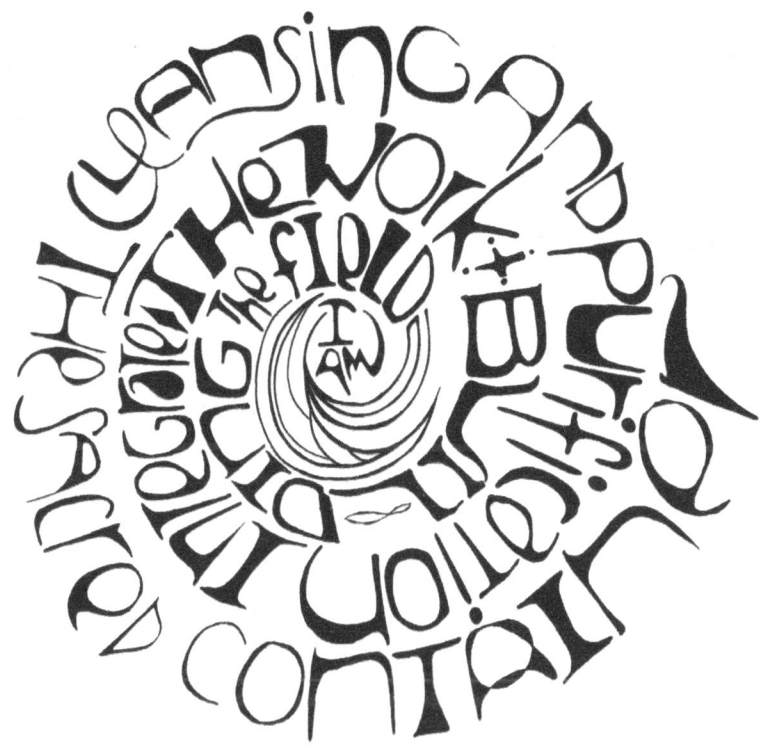

As you move through the six chapters, you will be guided to work on yourself. You can deepen your understanding and learn the details of the practices in The Healer's Process Practice Manual. Notations in this book guide you to specific practices in the practice manual. These are designed to be incorporated into healing sessions with others if you are called, but always start with yourself first.

Throughout this book, you will find various journaling prompts designed to encourage personal introspection. These reflections will uncover previously unknown aspects of yourself, laying a foundation for further exploration and self-discovery. Some prompts will guide you in healing emotional wounds and challenging core beliefs. Others will assist in establishing a clear purpose and motivation for your work. Additionally, some prompts will aid in articulating your services, allowing you to remain authentic and embrace success as a practitioner. Maintaining a journal and completing the prompts to the best of your ability is essential. By documenting your experiences, you can track your progress and discoveries.

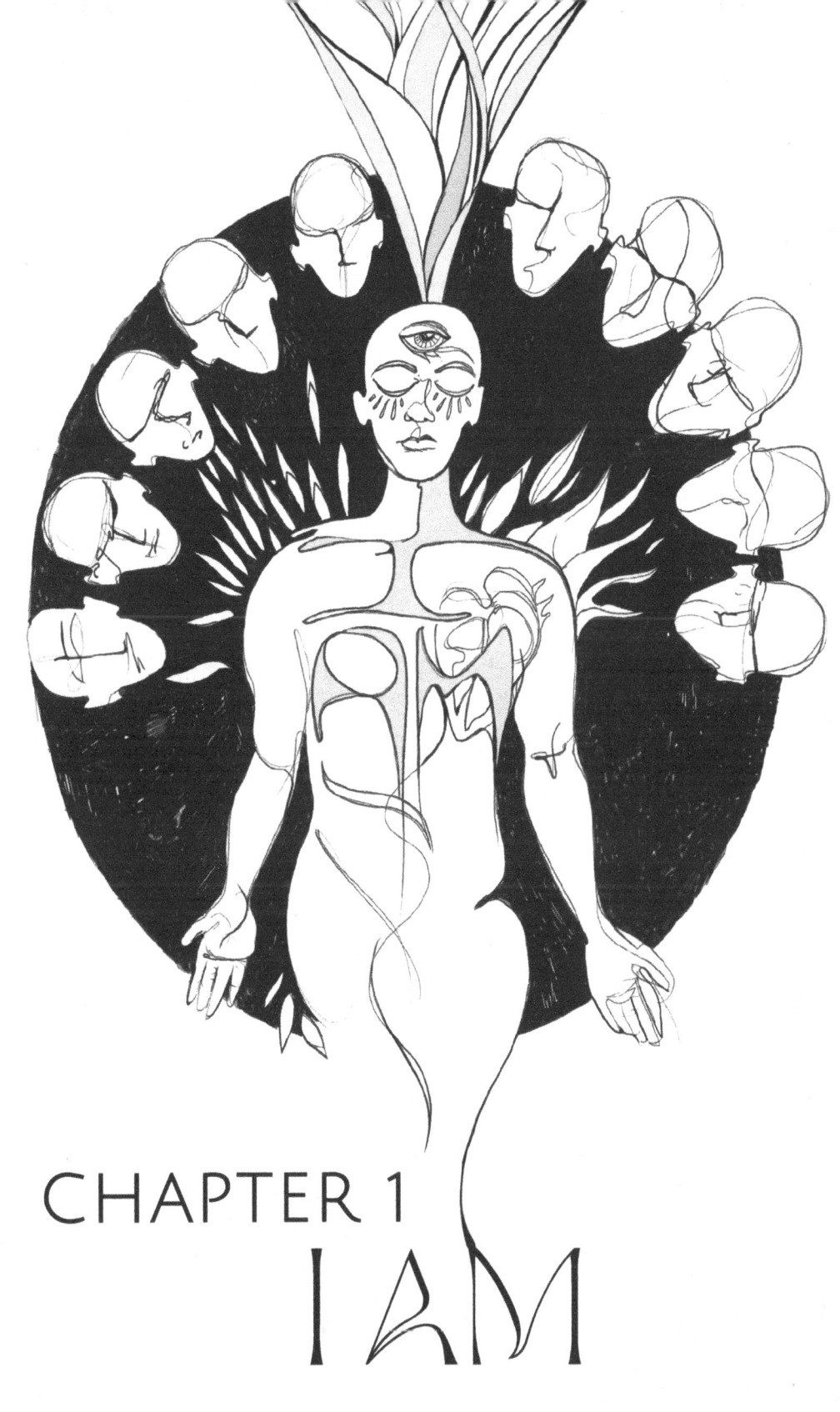

CHAPTER 1

I AM

CHAPTER 1

I AM

I AM is the longest chapter because it forms the energetic groundwork for your life as a healer and gives you an understanding of who you are at a fundamental level. Healers focus on service and supporting others, so you must build energetic power and resilience to sustain yourself long-term. Knowing who you are as a healer helps you avoid false starts, confusion, feeling overwhelmed, wasted energy, and dissatisfaction with your work over time.

This chapter will help you create a supportive personal practice, the cornerstone of any healer's life. You cannot skip these essential steps of knowing yourself, healing deeply held wounds and beliefs, and building your core of light and love. You must understand why you are called to this work, what it means to you, and what you are here to learn and heal for yourself through this calling.

The topics in this chapter include:

- You as a unique healer.

- Understanding, healing, and integrating the Healer Archetypes.

- Soul-level work and soul contracts, past lives, and irrational fears.

- Developing sovereignty, intentions, commitments, and devotions.

- Understanding and building your personal practice to the next level, breaking through resistance and fear.

- Understanding energetic anatomy and fundamentals of personal energy cultivation: building energetic power in the lower energy center and the core channel.

- Activating gratitude.

- Connecting to self, purpose, and path.

1

ACTIVATING YOUR 'I AM'

I am that I am.

Your "I AM" declares who you are in the world and embodies your wholeness. "I AM" are potent words; as you utilize them, you become more clear. You know yourself more deeply by the declarations you are willing to make.

Many people struggle to clearly state who they are, what they do, and what they stand for in their practice or life. When deeply connected to your "I AM," it reflects naturally out into the world, so you must make declarations that will carry you into service—"I AM" statements that align with your Divine truth and soul's code. As these are activated, you have the opportunity to shed previous identities and beliefs holding you back from your full expression. "I AM" activates the personal power of sovereignty. You, of your own free will, have decided to do this work and be of service.

As a healer, one of your most powerful tools is to witness someone in their wholeness and most advanced state. To do that, you need to observe yourself in that state. This is the "I AM" state of being. It encompasses all of who you are. It is your archetypal energies and core truths you've held for many lifetimes. In the "I AM" state, you are no longer hiding. You declare yourself so you can understand your healing gifts—not only from studying but also from remembering.

Your "I AM" statements will serve as a guiding light, carrying you forward and helping others find your medicine. They'll inform your inner awareness of your comfort and discomfort with aspects of yourself and your path, offering clues about internal work to explore in your practices.

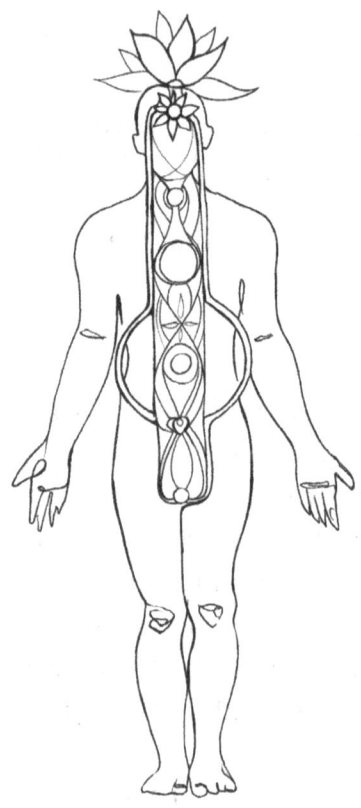

Central Channel

Your "I AM" is held at the core of your being. Energetically, the core is your central channel. This channel of light runs vertically through your body from the center of the crown of your head to the perineum, the center of the pelvic floor at the base of your torso. Working with this central energy channel cleans, activates, and aligns the energy centers along its path. Being aware of and meditating on this channel will center and guide you in alignment with your highest inner power source and wisdom.

When centered in this way, you will shed false, accumulated identities and find what you may otherwise search for outside yourself. You may be drawn to ask guides or other people for answers, but when you have activated your center, you will experience greater trust in your intuition and inner world. In the coming pages, you will be guided to explore the unseen realms and interact with beings. If you're not genuinely grounded in yourself and the Earth, you risk being knocked off balance and become lost in the external energies you encounter.

In Daoist alchemy, this central channel is called the "Taiji Pole" and is considered the sacred "Still Point of Humanity." This is where the energies of Heaven and Earth enter the body and flow to the organ systems. It is the home of the essence of the eternal soul and contains karmic-related illnesses and ancestral memories. It is through this area that we experience all change and transformation. It is also considered a magical gateway to the entire Universe.

Imagine this pole as a tube of brilliant white light in the center core of your body. In the tube, witness the flow of pulsing energy. With intention and imagination, you can move the energy, collect it in certain areas or energy centers, or direct it to specific organs. This is a stabilizing force for your energy, body, and life. Its energy radiates outward to create your field and feeds the physical, energetic, and spiritual bodies. Simple meditation on this pole will yield powerful results. Activate this channel by visualizing the light in the core getting brighter and more compressed on the inhale breath, while on the exhale breath, this light expands and radiates out in every direction. You will experience positive results by working with this regularly.

See *The Healer's Process Practice Manual*: [Practice 1: Activating the Central Channel]

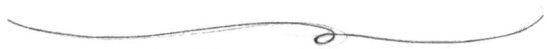

The Lower Dantian

The human body has three primary centers along the Taiji pole (central channel), storing energy. They are called the "Dantians." They are located in the head (Upper Dantian), the heart (Middle Dantian), and the lower abdomen (Lower Dantian). Dantian is from Daoism and means "elixir field"— where energy is gathered, stored, and transformed. Energy can be absorbed from your external environment, moved into the Dantians through the Taiji Pole, and stored in the Dantians, which act as reservoirs. It can then be distributed to the organs, energy field, and Taiji Pole. This energy can be cultivated and used for your health and well-being and to support your healing practice.

The Lower Dantian is the power at the belly button or just below (some say three-finger's breadth, but it is up to you to feel what is right for you) on the inside of the body, between the front and back. Think of this as your battery pack, as you'll be storing energy here for later. The corresponding concept in Japanese is *hara*, the sacral chakra or *Svadhisthana* in the yogic tradition. This is the seat of *Jing* (body essence) or *Prana* (life force), which radiates to the rest of your body. Focused awareness and breathing into this area builds power and helps you develop a clear "gut feeling." This is the intuition of your physical body, and cultivating your relationship with subtle signals from your body assists you in understanding what is happening internally for someone else. Connecting to and storing energy in this area helps you have more power in healing and not deplete yourself when working. This is because the natural energy flow from the Earth to your belly and through your body has been established and functions when you transmit energy to another.

The Middle Dantian in the heart gives you emotional awareness, empathic communication, and communication with your higher self. The Upper Dantian gives you psychic perceptions. All three bring a balanced, nurturing energy to your life and work, activating many layers of intuitive awareness.

It is vital to first work with and become robust in the Lower Dantian and then cultivate a balance of all three if you want your intuition, psychic awareness, or visions to be accurate and genuine. Many focus on opening the third eye or psychic vision before the foundational work of activating and cultivating the belly and heart centers. This can lead to physically and psychically disturbing energy deviations. This means that the energy is imbalanced in the body and even moving in the wrong direction, causing misperceptions, mental health issues, or physical illness.

A Lower Dantian practice will give an automatic starting and ending point, a place you come from and return to whenever you are doing a practice or engaging in healing work. Being practiced at returning to the Lower Dantian will support you if you are ever overwhelmed by energy or a spiritual encounter. You will not be tipped off balance by evolving experiences in the unseen realms. A simple way to begin this as a practice is to sit straight and put your mind's eye into your belly, feel the belly rise and fall, and imagine a light growing brighter with every breath.

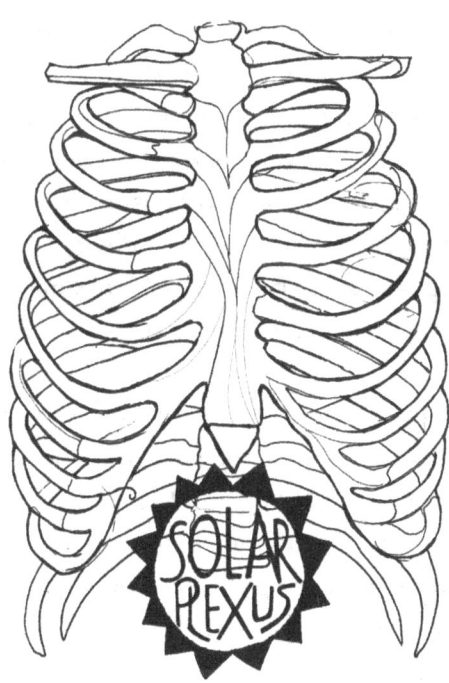

See *The Healer's Process Practice Manual*: [Practice 2: Lower Dantian Cultivation]

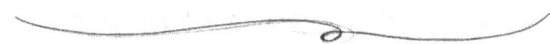

Sovereignty

Deeply connected to "I AM" is sovereignty—a state of genuine independent autonomy. Very few of us are familiar or comfortable with this state of being because shame and fear are used to make us conform and fit in, which creates an underlying energy of dependence and subjugation. Broken homes and social structures create anxious, codependent relationships. Addictions prevent us from being free and in control of our lives and life-force. We often need to engage in masking to maintain employment or acceptance by family or community.

This is why you must explore what holding the frequency of a sovereign being means to you and how you have given up your power as you actively choose to reclaim your sovereign state. Without this internal compass, you are more vulnerable to taking on others' energy and psychic and spiritual attacks. You cannot engage in the powerful invocation work needed to connect to light beings and guides without a clear connection to your free will. In healing work, you make statements and requests for the highest healing. Learning how to declare who you are and why you are here and ask for beneficial support to carry out your soul's mission is essential.

Within the confines of Western social structure, you might mistake sovereignty for non-connected independence without community or support. Here, you are developing sovereignty that is interdependent and connected to a healthy community of supportive spiritual and energetic systems and beings while standing in your own agency. You will see that being sovereign means intentionally engaging with what serves growth, well-being, and fulfillment.

In the quest to discover your most authentic medicine, you may come up against those who would rather you stay small or not rock the boat with your magic. If you are unclear about who you are and your self-governance, you might get distracted from or obstructed on your true path—maybe even for years.

See *The Healer's Process Practice Manual*: [Practice 3: Sovereignty I]

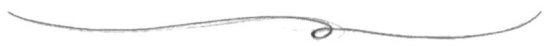

The Area Under the Heart and Its Relationship to Sovereignty

The area under the heart is considered the third energy center, or *Manipura* chakra in Yogic tradition. It is located in the area of the diaphragm under where your ribs come together—the solar plexus. When activated, this area has a radiant, yellow sun-like energy and is the primary center for your personal power, self-esteem, and self-image. It is also a collection point for repressed and unprocessed emotions. This center can become rigid, congested, and out of balance through lack of movement, poor breathing, overeating, and "stuffing down" your emotions. This area in Daoist tradition is called The Yellow Court. It is the court before the Emperor, the heart. Suppose your heart can't handle a situation's intensity, such as a significant trauma. In that case, this area is where repressed emotions and energies are held until you can process them. Complex and long-term trauma creates rigidity in the diaphragm and adhesions to the vagus nerve and psoas muscle group (the powerful muscles connecting the upper and lower bodies that activate during a flight or fight response), as the nervous system cannot fully process the repetitive stresses it has been managing. Many people experience a sensation that their energy is cut off or unable to flow through this area, resulting in a feeling that the upper and lower halves of the body aren't connected and communicating with each other. Working with this area frees up stagnant energies and emotions and allows energy to flow healthily throughout the system. You can begin to work with this area by moving your ribcage in spiraling motions, stretching your sidelines, twisting your torso, massaging and tapping the solar plexus area, and doing breathwork practices.

See *The Healer's Process Practice Manual*: [Practice 4: Sovereignty II]

JOURNAL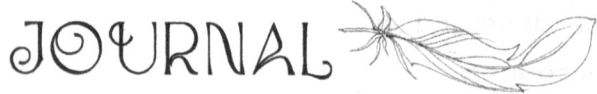

Answer the following questions:

- What has my relationship and understanding of my sovereignty been?

- In what ways do I sabotage my sovereign state?

- Do I engage in relationships in which I relinquish my identity?

- Do I put up with things against my highest good (especially from a desire to feel loved)?

2

COMFORTABLE WITH THE UNCOMFORTABLE

The only way out is through.

Healing is uncomfortable because it involves learning to feel instead of disassociating. Healing asks you to be in the body and experience sensations and emotions that have been challenging in the past. Negative beliefs and patterns are brought to light to be addressed, and early childhood relationships and traumas resurface in service to their clearing. It can be uncomfortable to reorganize a physical body into balance. It can be uncomfortable to lead someone to realize why they are ill, why their relationships fail, or why they are unsuccessful. Yet, these areas are where people need support and seek healing.

Sometimes, clients want to be "fixed" without being uncomfortable. As a result, they put up blocks to deeper work. They might rail against you, cancel appointments, or try to get out of sessions because they want to avoid feeling pain. Understanding this is part of the process allows you to show up powerfully, name it when you see it, and have the right encouragement for them to continue. You might think a client isn't showing up for the work because of something you are doing wrong, but they are responding to the uncomfortable experience of feeling new sensations and realizing fundamental changes are already in motion.

In this way, breakdowns become vital parts of breakthroughs. Breakdowns are uncomfortable, and most people shy away from or try to fix them instead of being with them in a way that supports healing. One of your jobs is to become comfortable with breakdowns, intense emotions, and darkness in its many forms.

Otherwise, you may misinterpret a critical process and push negativity deeper into the body instead of freeing it.

You've undoubtedly faced a challenge, and someone dismissed it or tried to change the subject. Maybe telling you, "It will all be okay," or "You are better off without it/them," or "Don't cry. It's not a big deal." These interactions confuse our nervous systems and shut us down. If this was a common way of dealing with emotions in your family of origin, you may have repressed, unheard, and misunderstood emotional residue in your system. This is common in our world, so you'll confront this type of conditioning as a healer.

I had a coaching practice focused on supporting men specifically. My work partner and I spent time helping men feel again, allowing them to access, track, and understand their feelings and how they could be expressed healthily. This was profoundly transformational work and much needed in a society that often shuts down healthy emotional male expression. We saw how opening these emotions was confusing and confronting, and releasing repressed anger and grief took time. But when a man who'd spent thirty years unable to cry texted that he was crying at the beauty of a sunset, we knew that this was an essential part of finding wholeness and peace.

The only way to prepare for "being in the uncomfortable" is to do your own work and lean into the uncomfortable parts of yourself. These are the places you don't want to touch, see, or feel. This means looking at your most hidden aspects, feeling (what sometimes feels like too much), clearing up old patterns, and shifting your energy to reflect the highest version of yourself. Sometimes, it might mean pushing yourself to speak, act, and put yourself in the public eye even when you don't want to be seen.

Your 'uncomfortable' may involve intensive healing from severe trauma, illness, or injury. You may experience mental health issues or frightening spiritual encounters. Many healers have been through great darkness and pain. You can't just throw love and light on your pain to mask it so you can try to be of service. Often, it isn't focusing on the light but looking at the shadow that creates healing.

If you focus only on light and positive thinking, you may miss deep, necessary work within yourself. You may ignore what must be dealt with, which will catch up to you eventually. If you cannot be with your shadows and pain, how can anyone trust you to be with theirs?

It may be that your design is all about bringing up these things in others as you wield the sword of truth—which isn't always appreciated or welcome. You might compare your work to others who are channeling light beings or doing other forms of healing work, which might seem, on the surface, easier than your path. You are important. We are going through a collective purging of shadow frequencies, which requires many of us to be present with these energies. It might sometimes feel like you are in the muck, but it is a very high service. We are also transmuting these shadows for our lineages and the collective. Through this, we do work that has significant global implications. People are moving enormous amounts of dense energy, and simply encountering you might bring it up. Maintaining your self-care protocols when in this challenging mode of service is especially essential.

Sometimes, we create discomfort and shadow when we are not doing our work in the world. When not fully activated in our leadership, we sometimes create chaos and drama to feel the discomfort we can naturally be present to as healers. I have met many with incredible natural talent. Yet, they seem to be constantly sidelined by emotionally intense relationships, unsupportive housing situations, ungrounded lifestyle choices, and community drama that seems to follow them around. Their choices keep them in a state of overwhelm, stress, and dysregulation as they process others' energy and emotions, try to stabilize untenable situations, and engage in toxic dynamics.

Your system and soul have a code to work with shadow. If you aren't doing that work, you may unconsciously create it for yourself. Strangely enough, this can create a binding cycle in which you feel that you can't be a healer because you have uncomfortable feelings and situations in your life, and they are there because you are not doing your work as a healer.

JOURNAL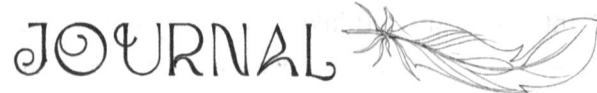

If you feel like you can't step into who you are as a healer because of instability in your life, ask:

- Am I creating instability to give myself something to work on?

- Is there an easier way to live, one that involves doing my soul's work and assisting others, bringing me a new level of stability and peace?

Shadow work, which explores the inner darkness, repressed, rejected, and traumatized aspects of self, is critical to personal development. We can also weaponize it against ourselves if we focus on it exclusively— forgetting other aspects of life. As the flagellants of old tortured themselves in the name of ridding their sins, we too can beat ourselves up with working on ourselves. We can become addicted to the emotional intensity of these works, always looking for the next layer of "what is wrong." Spiraling into pain and issues without allowing joy or grace. We can become lost in the shadows.

I had a client come to me after many months in the jungle on plant dietas. These restrictive diets focus on working with specific plant medicines along with regular Ayahuasca ceremonies. She had traveled to discover her depths but had dissociated from her body through the intensity of the experience. This extended time in almost total isolation had left her depleted and disconnected. She felt alone and full of pain, which, after such a long time of healing, left her feeling like a failure. She had put herself into so much physical distress that her underlying trauma couldn't be addressed. Still, instead of nurturing herself, she poked at her wounds by going straight back to her family of origin and living with those who had caused the initial traumas and pain. The path toward healing, in this case, was not more profound shadow work but food, rest, reconnection to self, getting back into the body, and slowly integrating what had been brought to the surface. Through stabilization and self-preservation, deeper work could be done over time.

It may be helpful to reflect upon the social programming of a Christian culture of original sin and martyrdom and how that might inform your viewpoints about the struggle of healing and shadow work. The point is not to suffer. The shadow is there to teach you, to encourage your growth, and to be loved and accepted as part of your nature so that it can be transformed. It isn't there to create chronic feelings of shame or brokenness. This requires a concerted effort toward balance. Play, rest, and connection with others help you not get stuck in your process so much that you forget the outside world. This can be an important reminder for your clients, who sometimes get stuck in this pattern. People need to receive permission to enjoy their life. Laughter, gratitude, and joy are some of the most healing energies to cultivate and work with.

3

YOU ARE A UNIQUE HEALER

Authenticity is a balm for yourself and others.

Y ou may or may not know you have a special gift, but you wouldn't be reading this book if that weren't true. Discovering and expressing your authentic medicine is deeply fulfilling and rewarding, but it is also one of the most challenging aspects of the healer's journey.

You may have a strong desire to explore healing and helping others, but you may not know where to focus as there are many paths. All have value, most have dogma and specific ideas about what it means to be a practitioner in that field, and each should create the possibility for your unique self to emerge. This isn't always the case. Maybe you have studied modalities to get practice, knowledge, and certifications. While powerful and helpful in many ways, these modalities can become restricting and sometimes fill you with more doubt than certainty or, even worse, more certainty than doubt. By this, I mean that many powerful practitioners have been trained from the flowing, inspired work they were designed to do into rigid boxes that others have created.

I am not saying that training isn't valuable. You need to know about the different bodies and systems and how to work with them for your and your client's safety. However, focusing too intensely on methodologies can sometimes prevent your authentic expressions. You may then set up your sessions, pricing, and business structure as your teacher did and spend a long time in that box wondering why it doesn't feel like the best work you could be doing or why you feel stuck, frustrated, and discouraged.

It's possible to spend a long time pursuing what others believe to be the right path. But what if following their path blocks the expression of the profound medicine you have held all along?

Use the following simple guidelines to break free of these patterns.

Listen to your body and gut: When taking in information from others, tune into your body and gut feelings. Test it out for yourself. People fall under the authority of spiritual gurus and guides and believe everything they say without question. Just because a text is channeled or someone has abilities doesn't mean the offering is for your highest good. Sometimes, it is a rabbit hole leading you away from personal expression and evolution. Someone may have a considerable following and speak powerful truths, but their work might not be what your soul is called towards.

Don't take all spiritual, energetic, and channeled teachings as scripture. The best way to swallow the false is to sandwich it between the truth and a profound spiritual point. A compelling meditation or healing practice isn't the end-all in these worlds. There are many influential teachers, those who have abilities and powerful exercises, leading people into cults or damaging works. Learn how to trust your instincts and inner knowing, and track your ability to feel into the truth of what you are exposing yourself to. If you come from a home where abuse or neglect occurred, where your thoughts and feelings were not acknowledged, believed, and held sacred, know that trusting your intuition might be more challenging for you. Time alone, time in nature, and exploring embodiment will help you trust your inner knowing. Always be willing to change your mind about someone and their teachings. If the teachings are solid, they will stand up to time and your questions.

Accept that you have done this for many lifetimes: What if you have already trained and developed, even taught this type of work, lifetime after lifetime? What if you are just supposed to remember?

Set a safe container and intention, and focus on getting out of your own way: Many force and follow specific protocols with everyone. When you open to the Divine, your guides and mentors on the spiritual planes, and your intuition, you allow a greater sense of play in your work. This could be taking a client on a walk or doing a physical activity instead of working on a table. Instead of hitting all the points from a protocol, dive deep into a particular area. There may be more talking, less talking, or sitting in silence. The way to find the unique expression of your work is to experiment and improvise, say yes to the moment, and sometimes try something you have never done before. This is, again, a practice of trust. Trust yourself, your channel, your guides, and your client's unique needs.

You are not your modality: Identifying too strongly with your modality can sometimes keep you stuck—only able to do certain work. People want healing and change, an outcome. Those outcomes are pretty simple. They want to get out of pain, have more and better sex, love, and relationships, connect to the Divine and themselves, have money and stability, creativity and expression, and look and feel better overall. Most of the time, they don't care how you get them there, only that you do. What is possible if you accept that people want to work with you, not just your modality?

You don't have to be perfect before you can help others: It's easy to think, "When I have figured everything out and have no more problems in any area of my life, then I will be a healer, coach, or teacher." Well, guess what? You will constantly be developing, growing, studying, and finding new and troubling ways your core wounds have tricked you into thinking they were gone. This is great! This teaches you how to access numerous tools to deal with these issues. It gives you compassion, context, and grace with your clients. You might still experience heartbreak, downtimes, illness, and breakdowns. That's okay; you are not a lousy practitioner or fraud. Get back up, dust yourself off, and get back to work on yourself so that you can bring your authentic expression to the world.

Don't be afraid to rock the boat and stand up and stand out for what you believe: Even if your opinion is unpopular, it might be the thing that saves others from a lot of struggle and pain. Part of your authentic healership might be going against what others say and forging a new path. If you have witnessed abuse or lack of integrity in a mentor or institution, it may be your path to stand up to those systems and develop new ways of supporting people. Maybe you have trained and worked in the Western medical system and realized it's failing our communities regarding ethical, accessible healthcare and education. Perhaps you were part of a spiritual community that failed to safeguard members' well-being. If it pisses you off, this is a good sign you are designed to do something about this issue. Consider what the more ethical, aligned, and healing way of being is and commit to that fully.

Be alone: Stop focusing outward and go in. You have the answers within you. Many seek approval from others over the inner work of learning to love and approve of themselves. Be courageous in your self-centeredness. This means being centered within your truth, light, love, and values. When you do this, you naturally discover what you want to focus on instead of "shoulds" from others that can hold you back.

Be in safe community: You don't have to do this all alone. Seek out supportive friendships that encourage your well-being and growth. Find people who like the same things as you. Notice when you feel calm and cared for and spend more time there. Healers are often lone wolves. We thrive with a lot of alone time, but a few close relationships with others on the path who can see you and love your magic are essential.

Follow your bliss: What inspired and interested you as a child? Explore, experiment, and play. Stop trying to get this right. Integrate all you are into your practice by incorporating art, dance, music, touch, laughter, crystals, hiking—who knows? Everything you have done up to this moment informs you as a practitioner. There are no limits. Things you were drawn to in the past can feed and specialize your work and brand, making you stand out and call in the specific people who want your unique medicine. This might feel uncomfortable. You might think you aren't enough in all your messiness and disjointed interests, but I've repeatedly seen people who follow their inner compass bring profound, unique magic to the world.

Bonus of Authenticity

Being authentic inspires others to be their authentic selves. You want to be of service; a profound way to do that is to be yourself. Around genuineness, people feel safer opening up, sharing, and being vulnerable. The most important aspect of the healing relationship has been established, and the modalities, training, and inspirations can flow through you in your unique way.

See *The Healer's Process Practice Manual:* [Practice 5: Unique Healer Declaration]

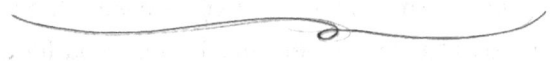

4

IMPOSTER SYNDROME

Some inner voices are to be illuminated. Others conquered.

Feeling like an imposter is one of the most common and chronically debilitating blocks of those called to the healer's path. One often feels alone in this universal experience. When you step more fully into your truth, an oppositional voice will arise. Each has a slightly different voice, but they come from the same places. They are structured from relentless societal conditioning that says you can't be special or magical. They anchor in from every religious teacher that ever informed you that the mystical, the Earth, and even your body's intuitive knowing are evil. They snuck in every time you were told you were weird. They arise from deep fears of your power, worth, and possibility. They are inherited and flow through lifetimes.

We are more powerful than we allow ourselves to be. The human race suffers from destructive codes. These codes are designed to keep us manipulatable and disconnected from the truth of what we are: creator beings capable of modifying the physical plane and manifesting a peaceful, just world. As long as we buy into these beliefs, we continue to invest in our suffering. We stifle life from flowing through us and creating beauty, joy, and healing. Cut off from our abilities, we live unfulfilled lives.

By taking up your place as a creator being and living your potential, you are actively removing this code from humanity and liberating us all. This isn't easy work because this is a collective disease. This is why I am guiding you to look at every belief and thought you feed as you deconstruct everything you have been taught about yourself, healing, and your ability to create significant change. You are a healer. Yet you may have a voice saying you aren't or shouldn't be. It will manipulate, demean, and sabotage you. Consider that you came to lift this code from humanity through your experience confronting this voice and telling it you are ready to step onto your path with all your focus and heart.

Find support by being in community with others on the path. Together, we build a resonant field you can contribute to and receive from. When the world doesn't understand you, you have to step into a new world. This is where you can share who you are and be offered reflection and care. Even if you haven't been exposed to them yet, there are others like you. Find at least one person to share your path and process with. More will emerge over time.

The voice doesn't go away immediately. It is a practice to confront it and drop its chains. Consistency and courage will be your friends as you shed your conditioned self and stand naked in the truth of who you are.

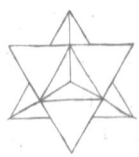

THERE IS A WITCH BURNING INSIDE OF ME

*She has been smoldering for years, waiting for the time
when I could fully handle her truth and knowledge.*

*She remembers the ways of the Earth's magic and all her creatures.
She remembers what it feels like to dance naked under a full moon,
pull a babe from a bleeding mother, and hold a sickly child through
the night, enchanting words of power over its sweaty brow.*

*She remembers how to mix the herbs, stoke the fire,
and tend to the animals when sick or dying.*

*She does not turn her back on the darkest aspects of life. She crawls
out of bed in the night to tend the bodies of the dead. She hears
the wails of the weak and the abused and comes to their aid.*

*Her pot is always on the fire; it is full of that which
nourishes both the body and the soul.*

*If I am to let her rise again, I have to accept that she rises
from and through the flames of hatred, fear, and horror.*

*I have to feel her burning flesh on a pyre built by her
own family, her friends, and her neighbors.*

I must feel her screaming through my blood and raging through my bones until I remember it all and accept that I am that witch. I hold her wisdom, her healing, and her power. But I also hold her pain, her fear, and her torture. If I am to walk the path again, the one in which I am called to be the healer, the mystic, the one in communion with the Earth, then I must own the pain of all of my siblings subjugated, condemned, and destroyed by those that fear nature's magic.

I must allow it to flow full tilt in screaming fury through my body to know her truth.

I must own all that I am.

A witch is burning inside of me.

Is she also burning inside of you?

When we fear to feel all of our past and all of our present, all of our sibling's pain and torment, we miss the power we hold as a lineage of magic people.

Don't be afraid. Her fire is here to bring you knowledge. She is rising again from the ashes; we have been chosen

to honor her through our bodies and our lives.

5

HEALER ARCHETYPES

The healer you are already is.

The word archetype is from the Greek words 'arche', which means 'primal,' and 'typos,' meaning 'imprint,' 'stamp,' or 'pattern.' Archetypes are the old or original patterns, models, types, or prime imprinters. They hold a universal energy or mythic character with fundamental motifs all can relate to. The archetypal patterning of human behavior is held in the collective unconscious, and our awareness of them is inherited and shared throughout all societies. They are expressed and interwoven in our symbology and mythologies. Archetypes are not merely inherited abstract ideas but living forces informing our modes of functioning. While they are connected to the collective wisdom of our species, each individual has their own personal experience of each archetype.

You hold many archetypes from all aspects of life, such as the warrior, the king, and the rebel. Some are stronger than others, and some are more activated at different times. In this section, you'll focus on the archetypes of the healer, exploring their aspects and their relationship to how you define yourself—your "I AM." You will uncover how the archetypes impel your actions, behaviors, perceptions, and emotions. They have the ability to renew your conscious life and propel you forward on your path, offering meaning, definition, and inspiration.

Through this inner examination, you will get to know yourself in new and profound ways. The archetypes will offer reflection points from which you can explore your unconscious, and their energies can bring strength, wisdom, and awareness. This awareness brings a deep personal understanding of your shadows and light or challenges and gifts. You can call upon and be present with rejected and misunderstood parts and step into your higher potential. Doing this work will enable you to awaken, explore, and heal aspects of yourself that you might be uncomfortable with and, in the process, self-actualize and gain power, clarity, and purpose. You will begin to access resources inherent in your own nature. When you deny your archetypal energies, those resources are diminished.

Archetypes are not to be defined by me but experienced by you. While common to all humans, you will have your own personal relationships to develop with each one. It is up to you to explore what emerges from within you. Archetype work activates what is dormant and helps you illuminate and develop what already exists within you. These inborn potentialities are always there. Left in the unconscious, they are capable of controlling or modifying your behaviors. You invite them forward to bring them into your conscious awareness and understand how they may affect you positively and negatively.

Your experience of an archetype may be challenging to place into words. It is pulled through the unconscious and altered by your consciousness as it rises up to meet you. You may relate to your archetypes through feelings and symbols, meaning images. This is the language they speak. You must then explore the depths of your own being to illuminate what these archetypes mean to you and how they are expressed in your life.

The archetypes meet you in the murky places between worlds. These are dreamscapes, imaginings, and creative expressions. So here is where you go to work with them. Explore your dreams, engage in active imagination, and dive into symbology through art - painting, sculpture, and music. This will help you integrate the conscious and unconscious aspects of self. You may want to receive a clear directive, but you will more likely receive a symbol or image that requires concentration, contemplation, writing, and creation to flush out its meaning. This is a powerful portal for exploration. You may want to overanalyze and intellectualize your experiences. It is a practice to simply let them be. Sit with images or fantasies that arise within you, and pay attention to them. Converse with them and allow them to speak to you in whatever form you can notice. Your work here is less about what you know and more about what you experience and feel.

Through this, you can examine unexamined aspects of being and develop maturity as you no longer operate and make decisions from unconscious driving forces. Your integrated archetypes allow you to express yourself more authentically. This authentic expression means you will be less likely to want to absorb other cultures and traditions to fill a void within. You will not feel that what is needed is outside of you, grasping at other's spiritual anchors, but show up to life with your own fullness and integrated self.

Your archetypes often correspond with your spirit guides. This means that if you have a strong connection to the shaman as an archetype, you will likely have shamans in the unseen realms guiding you. This is important to know because it helps you be aware to call upon those guides in your meditations and healing work.

You may be expressing a conscious or unconscious archetypal role in your community. Others will respond to these archetypal aspects of your being, and their personal relationship with that archetype is experienced through you. Personally, I have felt this expressed in how often people tell me they were afraid of me until they got to know me better. They experience me as scary because they unconsciously respond to the archetypal energies I express. Their own unexamined relationships with these archetypes are challenging them.

Healing the Healer Archetypes

Many of the healer archetypes are challenging for healers as well. We are aware of the risks of embodying someone who lives outside the village and doesn't follow the rules of the community. We have been societally programmed to fear witches and, even more so, to be accused of being a witch. As you explore your unconscious relationships with the healer archetypes, you will illuminate areas that you have been afraid of expressing. You will also begin to understand why you may feel so much resistance to aspects of yourself that feel strong and aligned.

Working with the archetypes is not something that you do once. They will interweave throughout your life, offering you growth and perspective. Your work with them will take you as far as you are willing to travel. You can begin simply by being with them and noticing what comes up for you. Because they are a part of your unconscious, you will have reactions to them. They invoke feelings that you translate into meaning. The archetypes may trigger you, bring up strong emotions, and challenge you. When you feel confronted, it means there is something to explore and learn. They may also make you feel expansive, powerful, or inspired. Images and feelings will emerge through your presence with them for you to explore.

In this simple exercise, you will begin your work with a healer archetype. Below is an extensive list to work with.

To find your dominant archetype(s):

1. Explore which ones bring up strong emotions or sensations in your body. Notice which ones you get images from when you consider them. You may also find that you dream about them or encounter them in meditation. Trust your intuition and use it as a guide to determine where your work lies.

2. Meet them fully by engaging in various ways. This can be through contemplation, concentration, imagination, writing, and conversing with them.

3. Explore the archetype's many facets. What have you been taught about them? What are collective beliefs and stories about this archetype? What do you consider their light and

shadow aspects? Journal to flush these out and then sit with how these aspects bring up feelings and sensations.

4. Embody, explore, and create personal connection through imagery, art, meditation, journaling, dress, altar-building, ritual, and objects.

5. Work with one at a time for the best results.

The Light and the Shadow

Every archetype has shadow and light. While the archetypes are not for me to define, I explore aspects of three healer archetypes below. This is so you can see how exploring the shadows and lights of an archetype from the collective and your personal unconscious can illuminate your challenges, blocks, or gifts. I offer a few key positive and negative aspects held in our collective awareness. Of course, each one has other traits that are not positive or negative. Remember that while a quality may be considered a shadow or a negative, it isn't "bad." When we label traits as "bad," we tend to push them away. Shadows are challenges. We learn a lot about ourselves and the world from our challenges, and they must be understood, accepted, and loved so that we can live a fully integrated life.

When considering an archetype, you may tend to focus only on its challenges and negative aspects. However, it is essential also to uncover the positive aspects and gifts associated with it. This will help you direct your energy and develop your skills. To fully embrace and tap into the archetype's higher aspects, pull the power from your lifetimes connected to this energy, and welcome corresponding guides and allies, you'll need to confront the challenging aspects. You can fully integrate the power and light as you heal your relationship with them.

Let's look at the positive (+) and negative (-) of the Healer, the Shaman, and the Oracle. Feel free to fill in others.

Healer

(+)	(-)
Spiritually, energetically, physically congruent	Leads to poverty
	Loneliness
Life of service to other people individually	Physical danger (witch burnings or demonization of healers)
Follows intuition	

Shaman

(+)	(-)
Able to move between worlds	Misunderstood
Spiritual warrior	Scary
Life of service to the community	Misuse of power/ ally with darkness
	Shaman (as a healer) would also hold: leads to poverty, loneliness, and spiritual danger

Oracle

(+)	(-)
Sees, knows, hears, and says	Being controlled (in the past by priests and rulers), so giving up power
Full access to wisdom and knowledge	
Service to the Kingdom (world)	Risk of being wrong or not believed, such as in the story of Cassandra in Greek mythology
	Lack of control over gifts

Fear of persecution, loneliness, and poverty

Notice the overlaps? Feel what rises to the surface when confronted with poverty, isolation, persecution, or lack of safety. Fear of the challenges can shut down your healing gifts or keep you from bringing your magic to the world. It creates stress and discomfort. These are often subconscious feelings that sabotage healers' lives. Working with the archetypes will bring these fears to your conscious awareness so that you can understand your underlying motivating influences and how to work with them instead of running from them or allowing them to rule your life unconsciously.

If they are kept in the unconscious, archetypes can live us instead of us living them. A fear of failure or expression associated with an archetype may sabotage your business or healing practice. Use your energy practices, movement, breath, and sound to move the challenging emotions of fear, rage, or terror out of your body. As there is a positive and a negative, the way to mitigate and control the negative is by enhancing the positive. Instead of being overly focused on the pain of being outside the societal system as a shamanic individual, focus on service, spiritual development, and practices.

Here is a list of some other healer archetypes for you to explore. Notice which ones make you uncomfortable, which cause a physical reaction such as hair standing up, sweat, or heat rising in your body, or which ones you gloss over as if you can't see them. Pick one to work with and use the tools above to explore.

Oracle, Seer, Shaman, Daka/Dakini Sexual Healer, Witch, Priest(ess), Therapist, Angelic Healer Sage, Magician, Sorcerer(ess), Medium, Guru, Nurse, Psychic, Mystic, Alchemist, Intuitive Healer, Sound Healer, Caregiver, Medicine Carrier, Channel, Midwife—birth/death, Earth Guardian, Past-life Healer, Mentor, Story/Song Carrier

See *The Healer's Process Practice Manual*: [Practice 6: Choosing Your Healer Archetypes]

See *The Healer's Process Practice Manual*: [Practice 7: Individual Archetype]

See *The Healer's Process Practice Manual*: [Practice 8: Pulling Down the Heavens]

JOURNAL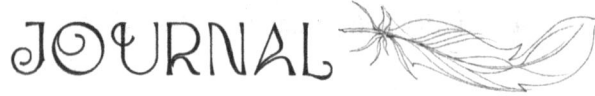

- What are the higher-level aspects of this archetype, its strengths and abilities?

- What are the challenges of this archetype?

- What about its place in history, or in my perception, causes me to fear taking on its power?

After you have journaled your thoughts and feelings, complete the following statement:

"I am afraid of integrating the [name of your archetype] because I fear [name the challenge]. If I am [archetype], it means that . . ."

Speak to your deepest and most irrational fears. Nothing is off-limits here. Here, you'll find significant, personal reasons not to want this energy, and perhaps why you are struggling with your path as a healer.

Past-life Experiences of These Energies

Often, your deepest and most irrational fears are tied to a residue of energy from a past-life experience embodying this archetype. For example, when free journaling or speaking aloud, you might come up against something that doesn't make logical sense, such as, "I am afraid to be an alchemist because I will be hung," or "I am afraid to be a medicine carrier because my family will be killed." These are specific fears you are not just pulling out of a book. When exploring, you might get a physical reaction, such as a burning sensation over the body or constriction around the neck. Strong emotions, such as grief or anger, might surface. These ancient traumas can keep you from integrating the archetype because of repression, fear, and soul contracts.

JOURNAL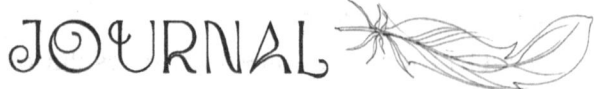

In meditation, ask to see, feel, and understand. Journal your answers:

- Why am I afraid of this archetype?

- Why do I feel triggered, angry, sad, or fearful?

Please allow me to heal what happened before.

It doesn't matter whether this is a past-life event or a story created by your subconscious to understand an aspect of yourself; the effect of the healing process will be the same as long as you see this as a way to understand yourself. Does it matter if your mind is making it up to illustrate something you need to understand and integrate or if it is a real thing that happened to you? Don't go too far down the rabbit hole arguing with your mind. Thank your mind for the input it is offering, and tell it that you are exploring something new, and please allow you to do so.

Awareness of past lives often releases stored memories, emotions, and energy. You might encounter this in meditations or dreams. Emotional release through crying, screaming, shaking, and fully embodied expression is beneficial to keep the energy moving and integrate your experiences. Working with these archetypes can, at times, radically shift your awareness of self and bring up a lot of grief or even rage. Don't be afraid of these emotions, sensations, and feelings. They are natural, and finding healthy ways to express them at home, in nature, or with a practitioner is essential. Connect to your breath and move your body intuitively as you go more deeply into the feelings and sensations. Connect your breathing and rhythmic movement to unstructured sound. Feel into the edges of what is comfortable. Allow the energies to dance you, perhaps bringing you to your knees, retching out what isn't serving, and then building you into a powerful expression of your full self.

If you move pain and uncomfortable emotions and sensations through your body, remember that they are moving through you. They are not you, and you are not them. Do not hold onto them tightly in an attempt to define yourself. As you move these ancient emotions and energies, you allow space for the knowledge and wisdom of these lifetimes to pour through you. That is much more the point of focus, not the pain that went with it.

The Wounded Healer

The Wounded Healer archetype, a term created by Carl Jung, deserves more attention as we all have a bit of this one. Jung contributed a lot to our current understanding of working with archetypes. He stated that an analyst is compelled to treat patients because of their own wounds. We are expanding this to include all forms of healers.

This idea has mythological origins in the immortal Chiron, a learned centaur (half-man, half-horse). The son of Chronus (fathered while Chronus was disguised as a horse), Chiron was abandoned by his mother. Apollo took the boy in and taught him healing and medicine. He was mortally wounded by a poisoned arrow and couldn't doctor himself back to health. Some versions of the story state that he supplied the poison to Hercules, who shot the fateful arrow. In some tellings, his immortality sentenced him to live forever with the constant pain of the unhealed wound.

This story shows that wounds can be pivotal in the healer's journey. They may instigate a desire to begin and strengthen your resolve to continue. Your wounds often inspire your inner journey to become who you are, and through great pain, strife, and personal transformation, you arise with wisdom and talent toward helping others.

A client's wounding has the potential to trigger a practitioner's wounding. To remain safe and in control, an unconscious practitioner may take on the role of a whole and perfect savior while the client takes on the shadow—wounded and broken with little hope of getting better. This is why it is vital to look at your relationship with the healing process and stay committed to uncovering your unconscious wounds and projections. Taking up this responsibility toward self-healing allows the practitioner to remain present and supportive throughout the healing process. Without this commitment to inner work, we might hurt those we seek to help.

> "A *good half of every treatment that probes at all deeply consists in the doctor's examining himself... it is his own hurt that gives a measure of his power to heal. This, and nothing else, is the meaning of the Greek myth of the wounded physician.*"

JUNG

quoted in Anthony Stevens, Jung (Oxford 1994) p. 110

Another similar story of the Wounded Healer archetype is Ọbalúayé, an Orisha (deity) from the Yoruba tradition, originating in West Africa. He was also abandoned by his mother and taken in by the Goddess of the Ocean, Yemanja, who taught him the ways of healing, and he became a master healer. A victim of scarring and leprosy, he covers his entire body in raffia, long dried grass. He is another healer who has gone through many hardships to know himself and heal the world.

While many wounds come from sources outside our control, others result from our unconscious relationship with who we are as healers or mystics. We can devise various ways to stay within wounded healer energy to the detriment of bringing our work to the world or creating harm inside our containers. Relentless self-honesty will illuminate your way as you heal the healer.

Sitting in inquiry with how your wounds affect your life and healing work can help you to:

- Find entry points to personal growth and further study.

- Give clues for your path.

- Inspire you to help others with the same issues or through what you have learned in your process.

- Find openings to vulnerability.

- Build community and resonance with others.

- Find deep acceptance, forgiveness, and gratitude for your wounds.

Experiencing gifts as wounds often holds healers back. Bemoaning your sensitivities and natural ways of relating to the world can become a significant life focus. You can see yourself as a victim of your innate talents and awakening gifts, focusing on them as challenges and weaknesses. Alternatively, you can become a functional contribution to this planet by developing a healthy relationship with them. This means honoring that you are sensitive and might need special consideration. Through this, you will learn how to care deeply for yourself and change your stories about being sensitive. These gifts, blessings, and superpowers may set you apart from the crowd but allow you to be the sacred purpose you are called to be.

Conversely, we can also use our gifts to separate ourselves. We become the savior and use our abilities to keep us from being vulnerable and connecting with others. We might become so invested in building our ego in this way that we set ourselves up for a fatal arrow to sabotage our work.

JOURNAL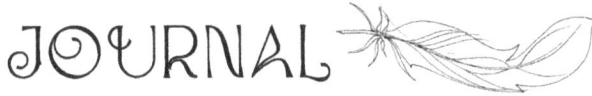

Look at the following list. What do you resonate with? Write more about that.

- I talk a lot about or focus on the challenges of my gifts.

- I don't care for myself first. I focus on others.

- I am fragile because of my sensitivity to shadows/dark energies.

- I lose sight of the fact that I "hold space" for healing and allow my clients to be wounded so that I can save or heal them.

- I want validation and reinforcement and attempt to control the healing.

- My boundaries are weak. I am pushy, or I over-give. I feel unappreciated or abused.

- I see myself as more special or separate from others because of my gifts.

- I use my gifts to show off.

- I don't let my gifts shine for fear that I might be showing off.

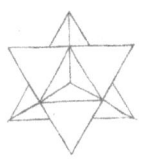

THE VISION

Spinning momentarily out of the trance I've
occupied for days, I see my feet.

They are dancing, moving of their own accord,
cracked, bruised, and bloodied.

Dust rises, coating my parched throat. Yet, still, I sing on and on.

In and out of altered space, I see the valley below. My
land, my home. How can tears still come?

I have danced and sang for days. I am the one responsible. I have
to save my people by appeasing the gods, the spirits, the ones
that have taught us and kept us in this valley for so long.

This is why I am. To heal and help, see into
others, and vision for the people.

But, this time, despite my dedication to the ways I
have learned, despite the lack of food, the dancing, and
singing until my throat is raw, I have failed.

I have failed.

My people are doomed.

We will all die.

6

SOUL CONTRACTS

Revoke contracts of the past that bind the present.

A soul contract is an agreement made at the soul level that can bind you for lifetimes. You might experience this as a significant hard-to-shift pattern that doesn't feel connected to this life. A vow of poverty, for example, is taken with the complete devotion of your being in a previous lifetime. You then find that making and holding onto money is a core struggle. Healers often hold soul contracts not to be who they were in a previous life because of the pain or trauma they experienced.

When one experiences a traumatic death, a soul contract can be written based on the event. This can mean any death that is violent, very painful, or significant because of its relationship to community, family, or spiritual or religious beliefs. Consider the masses of people who have experienced extreme trauma in witch and heretic burnings, crusades, and colonization. When death is accompanied by significant experiences such as torture and loss of loved ones and is associated with being a healer, mystic, witch, medicine holder, priestess, teacher, or leader, this soul contract can state that this activity or way of life will never happen again. This results in experiencing an irrational fear of being seen and known for these gifts. Inner turmoil arises from the opposing forces of your soul's code, your intrinsic nature as a healer, and the contract that seeks to dissociate you from that purpose.

You may be more powerful than you have ever thought. Maybe you were born into a restrictive family to hinder your capacity for magic because your soul fears expressing these long-known gifts.

To protect you from pain in this lifetime, your developmental environment and caregivers reinforce limiting beliefs, keeping the contract intact. Yet, your soul's primary coding (what is true beyond this contract) to be a sensitive, magical, intuitive healer is so powerful that you might be in deep internal conflict with fear, shame, doubt, and self-sabotage raging through your life for no apparent reason.

I want to share my experience of a soul contract in my life before explaining more about their creation and how to free yourself of any currently limiting your ability to step into your role.

The vision on the previous page is one I've had many times. I have wept and shaken with the weight and power of this lifetime, the one where I was counted on to save my community, and despite all of my efforts, they were lost. Writing these words chills my skin, even after years. At a pivotal moment of pain and suffering, the one that comes in visions now, I created a contract. I made a soul-level agreement never to sing, dance, or be a spiritual leader or healer again. Doing so would keep me safe and not risk a repetition of this heartbreaking failure.

In this life, I was told early on that I was tone-deaf and couldn't hold a note. This mild teasing wasn't meant to carry weight, but my child's mind took it in deeply. It was perfect—a perfect reinforcement of my soul contract. I wouldn't sing. I mouthed the words in church and even during birthday parties. As a theater student auditioning for a musical production, I froze despite years of stage work. Dance classes filled me with quiet terror. Born with a natural dancer's body, I panicked as a tiny ballerina twirling across the floor. In my twenties, I could only dance when using substances; even then, I felt anxious.

I was plagued with constant and debilitating throat infections from infancy. After an accident at twenty, my neck was a fragile place that made me feel unsafe as unpredictable flair-ups left me unable to move. The area of my throat and neck were vulnerable and challenged throughout my life until I went deeply into my work and discovered myself as a channel and one who sings songs of healing.

When my channel opened during my initial awakening, tones and songs emerged. At first, I shook with glottal stopping in my throat and diaphragm. Messages came in violent stops and starts. Expressing the strange phrases, syllables, songs, and chants was a great exertion. This was accompanied by visions—this lifetime of dancing and others as a healer in different ways.

As I began to offer my healing circles and the work I do now, I experienced overwhelming fear. It made no sense. It felt like, "I will die if I do this!" Yet, this was also my soul's code. I am a healer. I remember doing this work in many communities. I recall little houses outside villages, massive fires in the middle of a healing circle, and temple spaces where I worked.

I was internally divided and diametrically opposed. Knowing this was my work, but under contract to never do it again. I had to heal this, so I looked to the blocks and discomfort. My path led me to dance and sing. I forced myself to go to ecstatic dance, a free-form dance practice without substances or alcohol. The music has a rise and fall of intensity designed to invoke an ecstatic or trance state. Instead of dancing, I writhed on the floor, crying—my body in stabbing pain (for no reason). I felt as though I was being killed.

Slowly, I opened to heal myself as I chose to remember who I am. I asked for help understanding what was holding me back and how to address it in my practice. I was guided into pain. I processed fear. I cleared myself out with movement, breath, and sound. I saw exceptional practitioners. I allowed myself to accept my contracts and that I had the sovereignty to shift the agreements. As I did, I gained access and knowledge from the lifetimes I had been punished for being magic. I remembered how to transmute energies, mix herbs, work in ritual and ceremony, and channel my shamanic guides in my healing work. Through clearing past life contracts and their stuck energies and emotions and stepping into my sacred purpose, I transmuted the pain and fear stored inside my soul and body and healed deep-rooted pain, illness, and struggle. I sing and dance and declare and claim my medicine. I am free to be as I am.

Fearing Soul Work - Opposing Your True Soul's Code

My story isn't unique. Magic people are often conflicted because they want to help, heal, and do their soul's work, yet there is a powerful fear often of the "I am going to die" nature, so they keep getting stuck. It is inside the body, causing pain and disease.

When this inner conflict plagues you, it helps to heal the injury that inspired the contract. Yes, you can heal past life wounds. This is much the same as you would heal an injury or trauma from this lifetime. Through the process below, you might become aware of the story as a deep knowing or a vision, as well as an understanding of how this contract has controlled aspects of your life. Awareness of the story and realizing why you made that soul contract can sometimes be enough to clear the energy and illuminate your decision to free yourself from that binding contract. There are times when understanding the narrative living in your body will be helpful, and other times when you can become so attached to the narrative that you don't fully release the energy. Remember, you are choosing to reembody the true soul's code and release the contract. Knowing the story doesn't mean attaching your identity to it; retelling it repeatedly and holding onto the wound.

Death is a powerful portal. As a being moves through, it can create through intention, reinforced by a magnitude of emotional energy, a contract that anchors to the soul for hundreds or even thousands of years. This residue is what you are now clearing. Tuning to moments of death where these decisions were made can help you transmute the energy and rewrite the contract free of the baggage of the pain associated with this intense experience of the past.

While this might sound complicated to address, remember that you hold all of this information within you. First, declare your intention to uncover and understand what previously has been hidden. Speak aloud to your guides and yourself that you desire to heal these wounds and move past what has held you back. In your meditative practice, visualize moving through your past experiences and take yourself back to before you were born, into the space between lifetimes, and ask to be shown the moment when you have written a contract. When you begin to see, feel, or experience something significant, you can work with what you uncover.

The energy wants to be moved through the body system. Research states that when we experience trauma, a fight, flight, or freeze process is engaged, activating the nervous system. If we don't fully process the trauma by fighting, fleeing, or trembling (as needed even after a freeze reaction), this activated state can become stuck in the subtle and physical bodies. Even the soul is affected. We must allow this ancient trauma to move through us so the anchoring energy and emotions can be freed from the body. This can look from trembling to quite violent shaking, moaning, crying, and even screaming as the body releases the contracted stagnant energy. You may feel that opening this up leaves you feeling raw and sensitive. It might even inspire crying and emotional releases that last for some time. Know that when you are in this process, it is best to keep it flowing and allow the deep wells of grief to be expressed. The tears will pass when they are no longer needed.

This process helps break the contract. Adding a clear intention and request for support ensures better results.

Here is an example to open your work:

> "Guides, angels, beings of the light, and those that serve my (or this being's, if you are working with someone else) highest and best, I ask that the soul contract initiated at this trauma or moment of death be broken now in this and in all times and in all places. I ask that any and all information gathered in this lifetime that will serve the evolution and full expression of this soul's work in this world be brought through with grace and ease."

When you feel complete, thank your guides for all of the support you have received and send love throughout your timeline with an intention for healing to continue. From this clarity, write a new contract and state the sacred work you are doing in this lifetime to fill up the space of the old contract and create a powerful new intention and focus for your work.

I have broken this down more precisely in the Practice Manual.

See *The Healer's Process Practice Manual*: [Practice 9: Breaking a Soul Contract]

7

IRRATIONAL FEARS

The soul can fear what this lifetime hasn't experienced.

You have cleared fear with the contract work in the previous section, but now let's look at fear from another angle and how, by facing and working through your fear, you can step more fully into your "I AM."

You might have fear so powerful you can't get to the deeper layers to sort out its meaning, purpose, or how to work with it. You know something is in the way, but it is hard to figure out because it seems irrational. When something seems irrational, the rational mind will do its best to pretend that it doesn't exist. After all, it's irrational, so it must not be the real thing in the way, right? For example, it might seem hard to understand why you feel like you might die in a specific way, lose everything, or be rejected from society for following your path. However, when you look more closely at your irrational fears, you'll find opportunities to heal, grow, and claim your gifts, which otherwise might be missed. When you realize what's driving you, you can do the inner work to clear it.

JOURNAL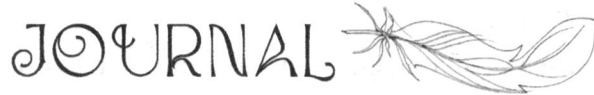

- What doesn't make any sense but is a very intense, powerful fear?

- Complete this sentence: "I don't allow my gifts to be used, seen, or known because I am afraid that [your fear]."

Going Deeper into Fear

Once you identify your fear, let yourself go into the most irrational thing that comes up. This could be a thought, belief, or strong sensation or feeling in the body. If you get a sensation, go as far into that sensation as possible, asking it to become stronger and asking what that sensation means. When you get something, be with it. Your mind might want to brush it away, but go deeper. It might look like the following example:

If that fear did come true, then what? Keep asking that question. For example: "I don't tell people I am a healer because...."

"I will not be taken seriously."

Then what?

"I will not be able to support myself."

Then what?

"I will die penniless and unloved."

That gives you something to work on, clear from your field, and invite healing toward. Being penniless and unloved has a powerful emotional charge resonating within the system, and any manifesting will be through that filter. So, even though you are trying very hard to do your work, this underlying block remains. This illuminates that you feel intrinsically unsafe to be a healer—a core issue and wound. Know that you can clear out what is hindering you from feeling safe on an energetic and emotional level and in your current environment. You now know you must focus on safety and building trust within yourself, especially in relation to your work. You should also focus on the lower energy centers, bringing your attention to and releasing tension held in the belly, hips, and legs. Cultivating energy in these areas will support your journey of embodying safety and trust in yourself and your work.

Keep asking, "Then what?" until you get to the most triggering, painful thing, seeking to get as specific as possible. When you reach the core, you might notice you are activated, overwhelmed, or feel dissociated. This can manifest as changes in breath, temperature, heart rate, or a spacey feeling. The fear you land on might make no sense, like being hanged or cast out. These fears, which have little chance of coming true, are often from a past life or inherited or cultural trauma or belief. Sometimes, it is enough to acknowledge the fear, feel the feelings around it, and develop a new story. You can also work with emerging energies through intuitive movement, breath, and sound. At other times, you'll need to do deeper past-life work. You can do this with a healer, past life regression therapist, shaman, or in plant medicine work.

You were born into a particular family, in a specific part of the world, at a level of income, and with certain physical traits that have given you access to aspects of yourself that wouldn't have been activated any other way. You have coded this life to provide you with a window into profound kindness, compassion, wisdom, information, and healing processes. Once again, what you have needed to find wholeness are the informants of the work you are to do in the world. You wouldn't seek out healing modalities, practices, and lifestyle changes otherwise.

Following a soul calling is the most challenging albeit rewarding thing you'll ever do. Most spend years avoiding and trying to figure out what the right thing to do is instead of what the soul truly wants.

8

THE HEALER'S PATH

Everything until now informs everything to come.

The two most powerful aspects of being a healer are your path and practice. We will explore the path in this section and practices in the next.

The healer's path is one of healing the self and then facilitating healing in others. Your path informs your type of healing work, offering clues you'll find in the darkest wounds you've had to heal and work through. These might also be the wounds of your family, lineage, or community and things you will have in common with your clients. Because you understand these wounds and traumas, you will have a connection to your people and can hold space for them as you embody deep compassion. This isn't to say that you're limited to a particular population segment or must have experienced something to help heal it in someone else. For example, if you have had to heal from sexual abuse, you have had to do work around the root and second chakra, trust, shame, and dissociation. That is a lot to know about. Pretty much anyone who has experienced trauma has dissociation to some degree, so this can give you information about your inroad to service. Your embodiment journey helps you track dissociation in clients and supports them in becoming more embodied through your presence and tools. Some of the best sexual healers have had to heal sexual trauma, and some of the best relationship coaches and therapists have had to work through incredibly challenging relationship dynamics. Had a hard time learning how to love yourself? What do you want to bet that teaching people about self-love will be at least some aspect of your work?

Beyond your wounds and struggles, your path has also led you through unique experiences, communities, educational opportunities, and careers. Many hear the call of the healer and wonder why they spent so many years studying or working in another field. Yet, if you contemplate that you have constantly been training for the present, you will see how your past informs your work, interests, and unique expression. When I was called to focus on being a healer, I was frustrated that I had spent many years and a lot of money training as an actor. On further reflection, I saw how my acting work was very shamanic and channeled and how that training helped me feel comfortable channeling in front of groups. I would have struggled with this leadership role if I had not trained my shy and sensitive self to be a bold, creative risk-taker.

You might think that you need to throw everything out and give up everything you have been to follow this path, but you can integrate all aspects as you develop into the unique blessing that you are.

Your path is a starting point of inquiry. The secret to finding your healing gifts is to pick up the breadcrumbs, the tiny messages that come to you—to listen and do the next small thing. Search for connections in your life. Find inspiration and awareness of your mastery through experience.

JOURNAL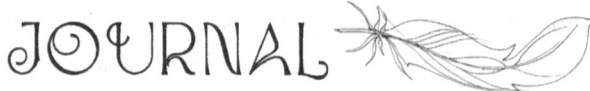

- What are the most significant wounds I have healed?

- What has created the greatest suffering in my life?

Remember, once we've healed something, we can forget that it was a part of who we are. We tend to discount or ignore the powerful work we have already accomplished. Often, we are not even conscious and aware of all the work we have done.

Go back through your life for each of these aspects and fill in your healing journey using the following headings to guide your journaling:

- Physical

- Mental

- Emotional

- Spiritual

- Sexual

- Relationships (including to self)

- Money and abundance

Write about your life's journey. Consider your greatest passions, interests, and natural gifts (even if you don't think they have anything to do with being a healer). Write about what you have learned and who you have become because of your experiences.

9

DAILY PRACTICES

Daily practice is your support system.

Your practices are daily rituals that hold up your path and often start or change when you need to heal. I am giving you powerful practices that will support your life and work, and it is your duty as someone on the path and supporting the paths of others to explore as much as possible. However, it's also essential to be guided by what interests you—is it yoga, Qigong, breathwork, drumming, dance, or mantra? We have access to so many wise teachers and different practices that we could spend all our lives learning and only skim the surface. However, your core practices should support you to:

- Clear and quiet the monkey mind and enhance your ability to be in the present moment and experience mindfulness.

- Move, challenge, strengthen, and loosen the physical body.

- Cultivate joy and inner peace.

- Connect to the spiritual realms.

- Instill a deep sense of grounded stability and connection to the Earth.

- Move unwanted energy (clearing trauma and stagnation). Cleansing practices.

- Cultivate, move, and build energy, aligning centers and nourishing organs. Purification practices.

- Create and maintain relationships with energies and beings.

- Give access to your intrinsic nature as a healer.

- Cultivate self-love, forgiveness, and gratitude for who you are because you truly know yourself.

Your practices are where you play, self-heal, and use your healing gifts and intentions to do healing for the collective. You develop a deep relationship with your energy system and body; through this, your healing gifts emerge, and your intuition blossoms. This time alone helps you access the answer to that strange mystery: "Is this mine or someone else's?" Daily check-ins make you aware of whether you are taking on others' energy or need to work on yourself.

Commitments to self-care, healing, inner development, and exploration are the greatest keys to success. It's easy to believe that more time on the computer, sitting and "working," or becoming certified in another modality is the answer. Some of the greatest successes I have seen are those who focused primarily on themselves and their practices, spent hours daily on internal work, and shared their experiences and what naturally arose through them.

I have met many healers called to the work who are disconnected from a commitment to personal practice. This is vital to your healing work's effect, evolution, and longevity. You are not separate from your practices. They are not for when you have time. They are the cornerstone of your business and life.

Consistent daily personal practice is essential. Morning practices begin the day with intention, and evening practices settle your spirit and prepare your body for rest. Cleansing and purification practices between clients keep you centered and effective. You will learn more about these practices soon.

Often, in this ridiculous world, there isn't much time for practice and self-care, and an hour or two in the morning isn't always achievable. I recommend doing the best you can to stay committed. It is less important to spend an hour for the sake of doing an hour than doing a focused thirty or even ten or five minutes. Don't beat yourself up for missed days or your practice not being perfect. Choose instead to give yourself positive reinforcement and praise for what you do. Acknowledge aspects you haven't seen as practice before. Taking baths, listening to music or meditations, walking in nature, journaling, stretching, and affirmations are all actions of important self-care.

Healing is an active journey that requires both movement and stillness. You need the Yin and Yang, passive and active. A daily morning practice calls in the masculine yang presence as the sun rises in power, energizing the day. You can begin from stillness and quiescence and then go toward active movement. An evening practice has a different feel. This is the more feminine, yin-flowing healing practice. It is done under the watchful love of the moon. Reverse the energetic order, start with more active movement and breath, and slow down to stillness.

I suggest committing to daily practice each morning and evening. At the least, schedule one evening practice a week. If this isn't possible due to family or other commitments, remember that all good relationships plan time for connection and intimacy; design that for yourself. Again, this is a case of being willing. Are you willing to take the uncomfortable step of declaring your needs and wants and building your life around them? These evening practices can be more luxurious because there isn't a full day ahead. This allows the body to enter a healing space where profound work can be done. Your system realizes it can go into an altered state and process the healing while you sleep.

Dive in deep. Allow the practice to take you where you most need to go. Then, take a cleansing salt bath, go to bed, and ask that the healing continue while you sleep. Before you sleep, you may want to declare aloud or silently: "May any healing I have begun for myself continue through my sleep, and may I wake rested and restored."

Mark these sessions on your calendar to hold yourself accountable—place reminders where you will see them. Keep tweaking your system until you find one that works for you.

The practices you enjoy and find most helpful will be those you can teach your clients. You empower your clients to heal themselves and spread these needed practices into the world. Transformation built on information alone goes in one ear and out the other or remains an object pondered by the mind. One based on feeling, movement, and integration through the physical body has a more significant impact and lasting success.

Avoiding Practice

When you or your client open your systems to deep healing, you might find yourself avoiding practice. You might become distracted even if you have a dedicated daily practice. Notice if you are finding anything to do but practice. These are often times when something is waiting to be uncovered near the surface. This also happens when you teach practices to clients, and they don't do them. They aren't lazy, insolent fools who don't listen to you. Deeper things are going on.

There have been times when I have found myself in severe avoidance of practice. I've cleaned my closet, watched Netflix, worked on my business, petted the cat, and found as many things as possible to get in the way of my practice. I teach practices. So what's it all about?

For me, these were times when I didn't want to feel, the times when my heart was too tender from a recent breakup or life event. I could feel myself needing to grieve yet not wanting to feel and move through the process. So, I avoided practice because, when I practice, I step into myself in a new, profound way. I listen, I watch, I feel. It is feeling that I am working to avoid. So, I will eat another slice of bread and butter, flip through social media, anything to keep from feeling.

This is the way many go through life. We can spend years avoiding personal practice so we don't have to feel pain, grief, anger, or shame. Anything ugly or that hurts. We can maintain it for a while. We might even think we are "doing the work" because we go to a yoga class or the gym, hire a business coach, or train in another modality.

We have a built-in system for avoiding pain. It is hardwired. So, you must go out of your way to grieve or work through stuck energy. The trouble is that the energy doesn't go anywhere without intentionally moving it. It buries itself deeper into tissues and organs. It weighs us down, and our physical health and well-being eventually suffer. These stagnant emotions and energies then attract more of the same. Other people spew their emotions and energy, which resonate with our repressed emotions. It feels terrible, and we chalk it up to being too sensitive and other people being too toxic. Those toxic people are there to signal us to do deep work. Once we have done this work, we no longer resonate, and others' energy and emotions can be witnessed without our taking it in or taking it personally.

I worked with a client who had lost her mother many years before. Years later, she was only beginning to unwind the grief and anger connected to this trauma. Pushing it down for so long caused illness in her body and physical pain and nausea to show up whenever she went into movement and breath practice. Through our work and her dedication, she opened up, let her body and the physical practices move the stuck energy into the light, and gave voice and acknowledgment to the pain. It hurt. It was uncomfortable. On the other side, she found the freedom and peace she had sought through other means but could never fully find.

As a child experiencing trauma and pain, you did the best you could with the tools you had at that age, even if the tools dissociated you from your body, shut you down, and encouraged you to hide. This taught you to hold onto pain as if it is the saving grace.

It isn't.

Moving through it is the saving grace. Allowing yourself to feel again can be overwhelming, especially at first, but freedom sits on the other side of feeling. You have to be ready, and some days you won't be. Don't punish yourself for those times or the time you feel you might have lost by not doing it sooner. You are right on track. You are unfolding in your way. Be easy on yourself. Start with the gentler practices that feel nurturing, even if that is a hot bath, a cup of tea, and a good cry.

The coping mechanisms and tools you used as a child will be the same ones you activate as an adult. You must learn new tools to shift your responses to the present challenges. These are developed in your practice.

Even in the struggle, commit to returning to your practice tomorrow, no matter what happens.

Practice Isn't the Point

It's hard for me to say, "Practice isn't the point" because I teach practice, where we heal ourselves and connect to Source. And yet, the practice isn't the destination. It is a vehicle to clear the mind, expand consciousness, and develop resiliency in this mad world. It trains your body for the intensity of light energy flowing undisturbed. It burns away the clogged gunk of life.

In our strange human minds, we are obsessed with latching onto dogma, processes, and systems. People have trouble participating in regular rituals or practices because there is an idea that they have to be perfect. Not the right time of day, the correct moon phase, the right candle or crystal available, the proper yoga gear, the time to sit for an hour, and so on can bind us into inaction. We use these excuses to beat ourselves up and stop ourselves from doing anything. Practice can be in a state of flow—anything can happen. Spirit calls, tools, and systems can be used with a heavy dose of inspiration and presence.

You may struggle with practice because you are neurodivergent and learning a system created for and taught by neurotypical people. You might be anxiety-prone or have ADHD and wonder why you keep losing your place in the practice. Acknowledge your differences with grace as you explore your unique ways of engaging with a practice.

Sitting still might not work for you right now. You might need a lot of movement to drop into that state of being. Focusing on music, letting your body tune into a gentle breeze to follow its flow, or watching birds eat seeds outside your window might be accessible and create beneficial results. Find the little things that work and follow those threads.

Questions to ask when going into practice:

- What does my body need at this moment?

- What is my soul trying to tell me?

- What feels good now?

- What is most present for me at this moment?

- Where is my breath?

In that exploration, there is space to find magic, heal, and deeply connect to Spirit. So, yes, have a practice. Devote yourself to it. Dive as deep as possible. Ingrain it so much in your body that there is no thought to it happening. It just is. Let it take on a life inside you and become a part of who you are. And then let it go, open to inspiration, and see what happens.

Truthfully, when I had no practices, when Spirit was purely leading me, I experienced incredible healing and shifts. When I had no idea what I was doing but surrendered to the moment, I did fantastical things with my body and soul. I had to give myself time and space to be deeply present with myself for this to happen, of course. From there, I had questions. I was unsure of myself. I experienced things beyond my comprehension, and I needed to know more. And in that search, I have seen innumerable other seekers. People travel from workshop to workshop, learn practices, ask for healing, try to figure it out, and are both served and constricted by practices and procedures.

Practice gives a starting point, focus, and discipline. It works. Your system, while served by the traditional practices, as all human forms are—of grounding, cultivation, storage, and flowing energy—is also unique and served by certain things more than others at certain times. There will be times in your life when running full tilt into the forest is the only way to go. There will be times when you most need to sit quietly and breathe into your belly. Sometimes, strength is required. Sometimes flexibility. Sometimes fire. Sometimes water.

Allow that the practice isn't the point. Develop such fine listening that you can hear and feel the answers to your questions and your body's needs at every moment. This is Divine inspiration moving through you. And far more the point.

10

THE AUTHENTIC HEALER

Stepping into your authentic "I AM."

Much of this journey begins with the powerful question, "Who am I?". As you receive clarity, it illuminates all the work needed for that to be your lived reality and truth in every moment. Your devotion to helping others calls for your highest alignment. Alignment isn't only about serving. It is about being a conduit for healing energy. You can't leave yourself out of the healing process. Self-discovery, awareness, and healing yourself will be guiding lights.

The medicine you bring culminates your soul's journey through pain, fear, and doubt, and bringing yourself into balance and wholeness. And that journey doesn't end. You don't have to be perfect to be a powerful healer. All people have challenges and pain. But, the calling brings you through the fire the quickest way possible (even if it seems like such a long journey), and that process begins and ends in the service you have to your self-development, your "I AM."

Helping others might be where you feel the most authentic, complete, and whole. You gracefully handle their trauma, pain, and intense stories. Yet, how are you at being held by others, your guides, and the Divine? So accustomed to being the giver, you must look at your ability to receive. So accustomed to being in service, you must confront when you cannot express or even identify your wants and needs in relationships. The path of the healer is one of healing yourself, which often requires learning how to receive, nurture, and advocate for yourself.

When you are drawn to these arts, they can't help but touch you. Calling in energies and making requests of guides and the Divine will change your life. There is no way around it. You might think you are working on someone and helping them heal, but you are also helping yourself heal in the process. If you are not doing regular work on yourself and receiving healing sessions from others, you may be suddenly confronted by your need to heal more profoundly. Perhaps a health crisis or breakdown emerges that requires sudden focus and attention. This might even knock you off your path as it teaches you profound lessons about yourself and healing. You might find illness, crisis, or pain as a doorway to receiving a new way of healing yourself, learning how to work with new energies, creating a new modality, or adding to your toolbox for the next evolution of your work.

While injury, illness, and aging are a part of everyone's life, challenges can be amplified by the residual energies you have absorbed in your work and not discharged. Your practices are where you can work energetically and emotionally to release anything you have picked up from others. These techniques will be explored in depth in the Cleansing and Purification chapter.

Challenges can also be wake-up calls informing you that you must live in alignment with your values. You may have unconsciously slid off your path by engaging in unethical behavior you rationalized at the time. You may have found ways of not being truthful with yourself or others.

Working with energy and beings instills great power, but power will enhance what is already present within you. Believing you can do no wrong puts you in danger of using your power to manipulate and influence others. If this happens, radical self-inquiry and counsel from those who can provide neutral feedback will bring you back to the authentic path when necessary.

There are particular areas where self-inquiry must continue throughout your career.

Ego and Judgment

This path asks you to look at yourself repeatedly and be radically honest with yourself. When gifts are strong, the ego can feed off that power. It can fool you into thinking that you are doing the best thing for someone when you are pushing them too far, not supporting them enough, or leading them down a road you think they should go down instead of what their soul asks them to experience. You are human; all humans have desire, anger, and fear. These aren't intrinsically bad, but your underlying motivations must be acknowledged and examined. Awakening gifts do not make those things disappear; they can amplify your most challenging traits while the ego fools you into thinking you have evolved past these baser aspects of self.

Your ego might push you into being too caught up in your client's progress, trying to micro-manage experiences to create a desired outcome. When you do this, you attach your worth to your client's progress. When they are doing great, you are doing great, but when they have a setback, you suffer because you tied your energy system to theirs. This is a way to burn out as you try to manage everyone else's experience. It can even negatively affect them when something comes up in your life. That is because of the cord you created. This creates co-dependence when your aim should be for your clients to outgrow you and move on when they are ready. They might still want to return for a new course, tune-up, or check-in as life or health challenges emerge, but they should not be stuck and reliant on you to feel good about themselves. If you are doing good work together, they will find that within.

Healing is about showing up, committing to the work, being present, and surrendering to the moment. If you try to control the experience or have a preconceived judgment about how the session will go, you lose the flow of energy that is supposed to come through. Preconceived notions and pre-judgments kill the surrender and spontaneity of the work.

Your client may not change, shift, or be cured as you think they should. This being is walking its own journey. They are living one life in a series of many. They came in with specific energies to transmute and have spent a lifetime or more building up disease in their system. You are not their savior. You are a guide. Clearing them of stuck energy and old trauma will serve them even if they leave this Earthly plane soon. You can lose sight of the larger picture of a soul's journey if you strain to fix and cure when the highest service may be to hold space for their process.

Judging Your Gifts

Another way judgment sabotages is by judging yourself and your gifts. This can be overly positive or overly negative. This stems from the illusion of separateness and our highly competitive society, which teaches us to be constantly in comparison.

JOURNAL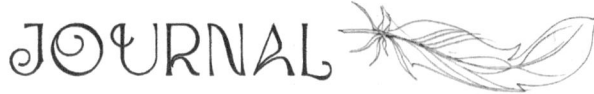

- Do I judge myself or others for "showing off," or being, or "too much"?

- Am I judging myself through this person as a mirror to stop myself from fully expressing who I am?

- Was I shamed as a child for being "too much" or showing off my intelligence, creativity, athleticism, or other gifts?

- Complete this sentence: "I *don't* want to be . . . because if I am, I will . . ."

For example: "I *don't* want to be too much. Something terrible will happen if I am too much, too powerful, or big." This often comes with, "If I am who I am, I will not be loved, have a partner, have friends, or I will lose my community, current clients, job, etc."

You must look at everything that keeps you from being who you are and being seen. Pay attention to internal judgments of what you don't or can't do and the words you use to describe yourself. I told myself and others for years that I didn't see things psychically. I judged myself by comparing my experience to friends with sight as a significant component of their work. I would imagine their experience and compare mine to this made-up reality. I judged myself and then made statements about it, which would reinforce my experience. I began to see more when I acknowledged what I saw. When I use the phrase, "I see.." or "It looks like.." images rush in. They are not often like looking at a picture, but as though I know an image. Gifts must be acknowledged, appreciated, and worked with.

JOURNAL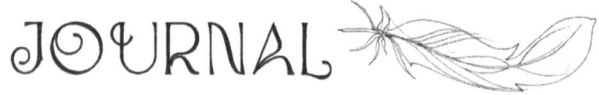

Look at each gift or ability and how it triggers you. Do you have a belief about being unable to access one of these areas of psychic awareness? Do you have an old story around these that keeps you stuck? Are you afraid of accessing one or more of these abilities? What fears come up? What is uncomfortable or overwhelming about what you (or how you have in the past):

- See (psychic vision)

- Feel (sensational awareness of information)

- Know (deep knowing for no reason)

- Hear (inner or external voices or sounds)

- Smell (experiencing aromas that others can't)

- Taste (getting tastes that bring information)

- Dream (heightened dream states or lucid dreaming)

- Travel To (astral traveling or journey work)

- Speak (able to bring through wisdom as you speak... channeling)

- Other

- For example:

- "It is uncomfortable that I know things because if I know

things that will put people off, they won't like me."

- "I have dreams that come true, and that scares me because what if I dream something bad will happen, and I can't stop it?"

- "I don't like seeing things because it scared me as a child, or my parents told me to stop doing it."

Once you are aware of the beliefs and stories hiding behind your gifts, you can consciously choose to engage with them differently. Try on new ones, make more empowered statements, and offer to the parts of you that feel scared or ashamed that they are safe and you hear them and love them. You can follow that up with, "It's okay to see, feel, know, etc. I am safe, and no one will be mad at me or hurt me. It is safe to be seen. It is safe to be seen."

If that brings up energy or emotions in your body, breathe to move them through, shake, and make sounds as you allow the energy to dissipate into the Earth. End with placing your hands on your body, soothing yourself, and feeling your embodied presence.

Your authentic healership asks you to go deeply into yourself. It is a courageous journey of exploration and transmutation as deepening layers of devotion unfold. Through self-work, reflection, and support, you'll find a fulfilling path, as it constantly evolves and offers you glimpses of light, love, healing, and creation you never knew were possible.

11

GRATITUDE

Gratitude is the primary key of the healer's path.

W orking from the space of gratitude is the most common thread of all healers and indigenous communities throughout history. Gratitude is a mindset, a conviction that always occupies your consciousness. It is an embodied experience that nurtures and expresses. Because it is a fundamental shift in your being, it must be practiced to be integrated fully. It is powerful because it is so personally authentic. It is the Divine language that the Holy receives and opens communication with the other realms.

Meditate on and write your gratitudes daily as a powerful practice. Speak them out loud and sing them. Even if you don't have a good relationship with your voice, speak aloud in your practices and tone and sing daily. All humans can sing. Realize that if you are committed to healing and being healed, you must work on all aspects of yourself, your voice included.

A gratitude practice is essential for opening a session or the day. It keeps the energy flowing and your heart activated. Express your deep, heartfelt gratitude for all that is, for abundance, for help and guidance, and for the opportunity to do this powerful work and be of service to the world. You might say: "Thank you. Thank you. Thank you. Thank you. I am so grateful for all of my life's blessings and my calling into this service. I am so grateful to be able to do this work today and for the opportunity to be a channel of healing and transformation."

Gratitude sets the stage for helper guides and spirits to find inspiration in assisting you. After all, you are creating a feedback loop with positive energies. Gratitude connects you to what is truly important and allows you to be present to the beauty of life. Deep reverence and gratitude shift negative moods, tiredness, and lack of focus. Gratitude brings you into the present and opens your heart.

A gratitude practice can take as long as you like. It can change and evolve every time you do it. It can be fun, whimsical, and full of joy. It can be profoundly connected to your heart and soul and might bring tears when you realize how deeply you feel. The more you feel gratitude, the deeper your healing will become. The sense of grabbing and trying to control the session falls away as it becomes more and more apparent that every moment is a blessing and that whatever happens in the healing is perfect.

For example: "Thank you, thank you, thank you, thank you. Thank you, thank you, thank you, thank you. I am so grateful for all that I have and all that I am. Thank you for the abundance that flows through my life and my connection to all beings. I am so grateful to be allowed to do this powerful work and be assisted on this path of healing. I am grateful for my family, dear friends, and all those who show up for healing and transformation. I am grateful for the service I am in the world, and I show up fully every moment. I am grateful for the food that sustains my body, my home, and all the comforts I am blessed to enjoy. Thank you for the continued assistance and guidance toward my highest and best."

This practice draws you into pure gratitude for all you are and have. Do this before a client shows up, in some way at the end of the session to help anchor these frequencies for them, and after they leave.

Gratitude connects the Divine, Earth, and self. This world is often overwhelming. You may feel you can't manage the number of clients (or stress from lack of clients) or the amount of work, networking, or social media engagement required for success. Gratitude helps you not feel so overwhelmed. It allows you to enter your work in a high vibration to deal with people who have emotional and physical issues, trauma, entities, or anything else.

Gratitude raises your vibration instantly. Nothing of a lower vibration can enter that of a higher vibration. So, it is an additional protective field. Gratitude for healing gifts, clients, abundance, mentors, and teachers helps draw these things toward you, even if you don't feel they are in your field yet.

JOURNAL

Make a list of what you are grateful for. Speak, write, and sing your gratitude. Repeat daily.

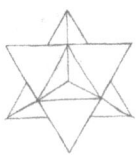

WITH GRATITUDE AND GRACE

With gratitude and grace, I accept my path here in this lifetime.

I allow growth and transformation to enter so that I might ever be able to better serve and hold space for change and healing.

I accept massive help from my guides and the beings of light who are here for my highest and best.

I vow to show up, be present, and share my gifts.

I ask for help and receive it from my powerful friends and teachers.

I dance at my limits and encourage you to meet yours.

I allow you to see me. Vulnerable. Free.

12

YOUR CORE WHY—INTENTION, COMMITMENT, AND DEVOTION

*To fully step into your "I AM," you must
know why you are doing this work.*

A clear why and understanding of your intentions, commitments, and devotions will help you move through all the other stuff associated with being a healer in the modern world. Gone are the days of receiving a chicken for healing. Gone are the days of being in a community where your purpose was the only thing you had to do daily. You must also do computer work, marketing, administration, and taxes. You know, the things that make you want to give up and get a "real" job. Your Core Why keeps you going and excited about what you are doing. It brings up an emotional response that infuses your actions.

JOURNAL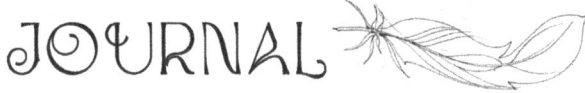

Take a few moments to imagine the world you live in, the people around you, and society.

- What would you love to see changed?

- What are you passionate about?

- What do you love contributing?

- What possibilities for humanity inspire you?

Write as much as you can. Then, notice common threads and craft a single statement to succinctly focus your Core Why into being. Remember, this may shift and change over time. I encourage you to revisit this often. I hang mine on the wall near my desk.

Here is an example of my Core Why: "I do this work so that all people are free to be fully expressed, magical, whole, and healed, no longer medicating, and can access higher consciousness and wisdom. Through this, we globally shift environmental and social crises and push through humanity's radical evolution!"

Intention, Commitment, and Devotion

The path we walk requires continuous declarations of intentions and commitments and then action follow-through in the form of devotion.

You set your intention as the aim of your Core Why becoming manifest. You intend to experience the outcome of your Core Why as reality in your lifetime. You are setting your purpose and target for your efforts. The commitment is how you will show up. It is a declaration of follow-through toward that intention. It is a contract that seals in your focus on this path. From both of those is born devotion. Devotions are the actions you take to get you there.

I will guide you to clarity on these through the journaling exercise below, but first, let's illuminate these concepts further.

Intentions, Commitments, and Devotions Feed Each Other and Support You

Intentions, commitments, and devotions are guiding winds that keep you going in a specific direction. Life's richness expands as every action leads you where you want to go, and aspects of your life that are not aligned fall away with more ease.

Intention brings meaning to the path. You aren't doing healing work just because you have some gifts and skills. You have a beautiful, illuminating dream that calls you forward. A grain of rice eaten with the intention of a ceremony is a ceremony. You can eat a bowl of rice in a meaningless way. So, too, you can go through your entire day without awareness of your intentions and live a less "on purpose" life.

Intention is also crucial in your healing work. The more intentional you are, the more effective your work becomes. Heightened intention transforms your practice and cuts down on how "hard" you have to work. The guiding light of the highest of healings already being here draws you and your client forward, informing emergent, creative work. Lack of intention can cause you to lean on modality and protocol as you focus on what you're doing to a client instead of listening to what is most present and allowing that to guide you. There is a tendency to be repetitive and stagnant instead of allowing unfolding inspiration. You might prioritize doing over being. Your beingness is a considerable part of the medicine you hold.

Commitment is your resolve. It is your stake in the ground to fulfill your sacred purpose. Even when you struggle, you can tune into your commitment and see where you are going. You are claiming your path and why you are here.

Devotions are your daily actions and practices that bring your intention to reality through the focus of your commitment. You step into your purpose as a devotee. Your work becomes a sacred temple where you come to offer and pray. Your actions become beautiful rituals and ceremonies. It is a prayer when you are uncomfortable in your practice and an expression of your devotion.

Devotion gives you access to a new relationship with discipline. Shift your mindset from thinking of discipline as hard, tedious, or something imposed upon you to an expression of devoted love.

Your personal growth and expansion of your service arise from clear intentions backed up by firm commitments. These commitments inspire your actions of devotion and discipline as you create the world you know is possible.

When connected to this cycle, you'll have access to something that keeps you going when you don't want to get out of bed to write a newsletter, post on social media, or do your practice. Have you noticed that doing something for yourself sometimes doesn't feel like enough of a reason? Many caretakers can't be bothered with self-care until they realize it would benefit how their children or partners care for themselves. Others are inspired if they know it will positively impact their clients or community. You might have to shift your focus to the larger picture of what you are here to do and accomplish. Sustaining inspiration bolsters you even through challenges.

I am writing this book not just because I want to write a book. I can (and have) put off working on it for months. When I focus on producing what I needed to advance on my path, I am inspired and present to the task. By empowering more healers than I can work with one-on-one, I have the opportunity to fulfill my Core Why and create a significant impact.

Commitments, intentions, and devotions feed each other. The more you devote to your practices, the clearer your intentions, and the more you commit, the easier it is to do the practices.

JOURNAL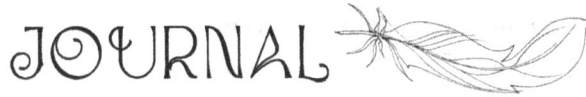

- What do you intend?

- What do you commit to?

- What are you devoted to?

Now complete this statement: "I intend for [insert your desired intention], so I *commit to* [*insert your commitment*]. And because of this firm commitment, I can devote myself to [insert what you can devote yourself to]."

For example: "In writing this book, I intend to bring you into greater alignment with your healing gifts and path. I commit to showing up as I write with the fullness of my being, my whole heart, and the presence of my soul. I commit to offering healing and wisdom. I devote myself to being communicative, open, authentic, and honest. I devote myself to my self-care, further study, and training. I devote myself to doing my inner work, study, and reflection. I devote myself to regular writing."

When you get clear, write them down, put them where you can see them, and state them out loud regularly. Remember the power of your spoken words as they weave reality. When you return to these phrases, honor yourself for being in alignment, or ask yourself, "What would help me be more aligned with these statements today?"

Be clear and concise. Speak with authority and power. Use your full voice as much as possible. You are calling your future to meet you now. As you get used to speaking these out loud, it will help you state your mission and offerings easily to others. Your inspired connection to your work is an invitation to those who seek your medicine.

You are also inviting guides and beings to support you. Spiritual forces assess your level of commitment, honoring where you are and what you can show up for. The more committed you are to the path, the more assistance you'll be given. They must be invited to your work just as you invite clients. If you believe what you say, the spiritual and the mundane will show up for you.

13

YOUR STORY MATTERS

Where have you been, who are you, and who are you becoming?

Sharing your truth, purpose, and mission (Core Why) draws people toward you. Allowing people to witness your commitments and devotions offers an intimate awareness of your driving forces, values, and principles. People want to know the person they see for healing work. They want connection, which helps them trust you and what you bring.

When you are more authentic and open and outing yourself to the public, you will hit up against fear—everyone does. You might be afraid that you will lose love and acceptance or that people will judge you. These natural fears arise from vulnerability, and expressing your truth and magic is vulnerable. While some people may judge or even reject you, there will be 10, 20, or 100 people to take their place. Your journey and story will significantly heal people who deeply resonate with you. These are your people.

I've worked with many successful people who have suddenly felt called to do deeper, energetic, shamanic, and spiritual work. They always fear their current clients will shun them, and their business will tank. They have been pleasantly surprised to discover that this is what their people have been waiting for!

As I've said, being your authentic "I AM" permits others to do the same—healing in and of itself. People yearn for realness to relate to. We live in a time of social media, where people become famous with facades of perfection. The perfect angle, good lighting, and a skilled surgeon can accomplish a lot. This fools us, but only up to a certain point.

You might think you should look like you've always had and have it all together to have authority and get clients. Being real gives you authority and evokes trust. Think of Brene Brown and her captivating talks about vulnerability and shame. Would we eat up everything she was saying if she wasn't taking us through her uncomfortable personal process? Let others see you've had wounds and been through the fire (if that is the case). You have earned the tools and wisdom to support them. You don't have to be perfect all the time. Be human. Show up vulnerable, open, and present; they will trust you. Trust is the cornerstone of a healing relationship. If someone trusts you, they will dive into their process more quickly and be willing to follow your coaching and advice.

If you choose to hide instead and create a facade, you must maintain it. You are, eventually, lying to everyone, even yourself.

I AM Closing

As we close the "I AM," I hope you feel your core solid and your purpose shining. Come back to the concepts and practices in the "I AM" to recenter yourself and explore other aspects of your healer's path as they emerge.

We will build on what you have learned in this chapter in the rest of the book.

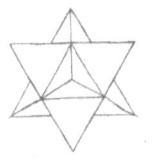

YOU ARE MAGIC

Will you accept it?

You are a bridge brought to hold the way for the light.

*Move toward the part of yourself that is certain
of the truth—your deep knowing.*

*Your expression of magic is entirely unique. You are a shining
dewdrop on the web of light, spun to link our consciousnesses.
This web ensures that the work we do for one benefits all.*

*When you rise in the calling of the light, you are allowed to witness
yourself as the Divine being that you are and have always been.*

You are magic. You have simply forgotten the truth.

Magic is your birthright.

Magic is your soul, crying to be set free.

*Owning your magic means trusting and accepting the
differences that set you apart and make you whole.*

*Magic asks you to receive your guidance from Spirit and
surrender to more and more authentic ways of being.*

*I'm afraid, at a certain point, you can't go
back. It will propel you forward.*

It has its own mission and power. Resistance creates dis-harmony.

Responsibility comes with accepting that you are magic.

*This responsibility is to shine. It is to clear out what
is in the way of magic being expressed.*

It means holding space for the light to shine in others.

You are magic. Will you accept it?

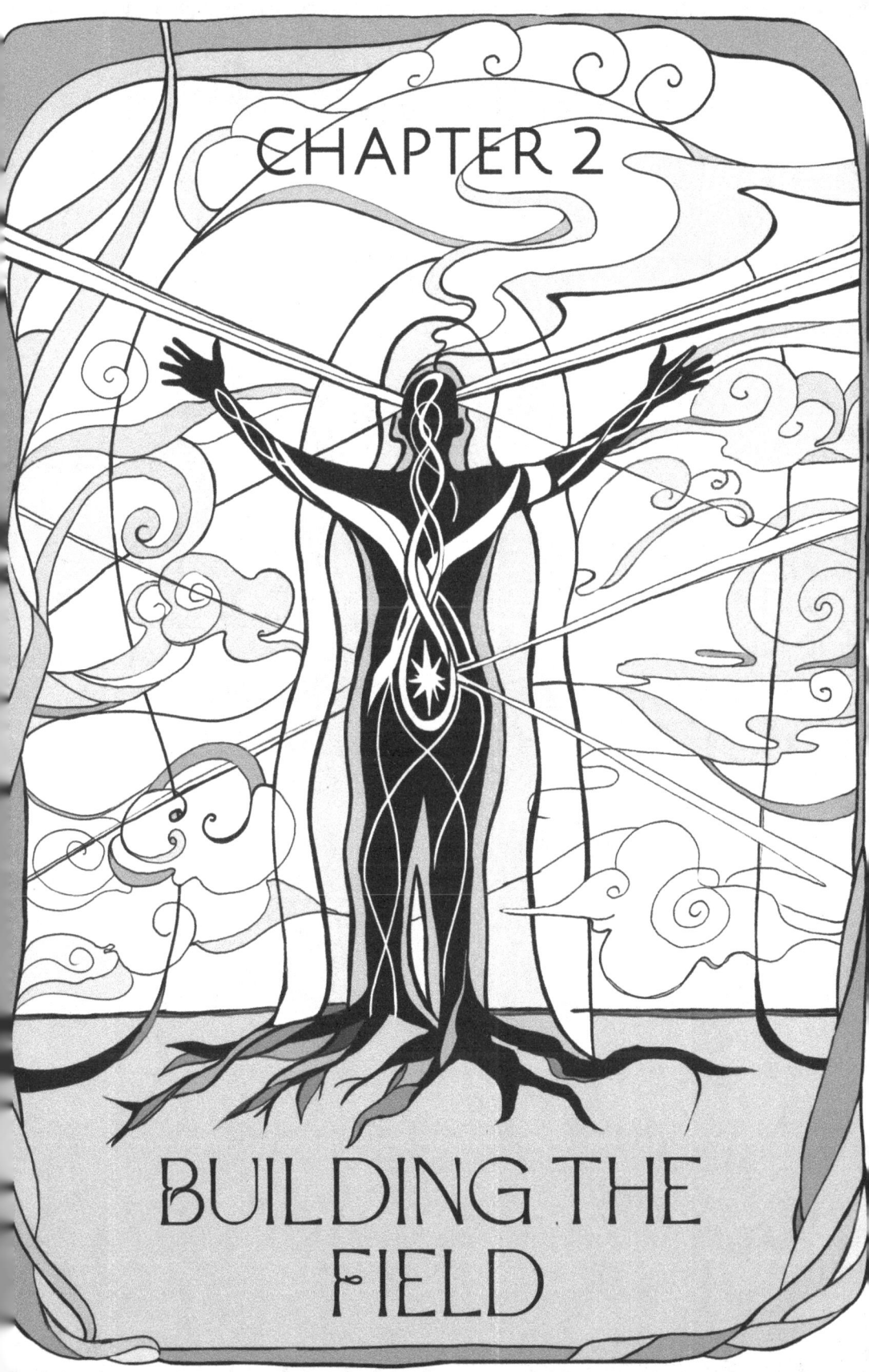

CHAPTER 2

BUILDING THE
FIELD

CHAPTER 2

BUILDING THE FIELD

The next step in your journey involves building your field. You are transitioning from an inward focus at the core of your being to expanding your focus outward into your energetic bubble or cocoon surrounding your body. This field is the unseen (for most people) energy body, an extension of you beyond the physical. Your field has many layers, and later, you will learn about them and how they constantly communicate with your energy centers, central channel, and physical, emotional, mental, and spiritual bodies and systems. As I teach about these different fields, I will use the plural, and sometimes I will say field to represent their totality. This chapter will help you understand how your field and energy centers work and their interactions with energy and the outside world. You will learn how to cultivate energy from the earth and the divine to become a more radiant presence. Through this, you will discover how your field dictates your life experiences and how to work with the field in healing.

No matter how good your modality, you must maintain a core resonance of light (your central channel work in the first chapter) and know how to cultivate energy to build your protective field. This field interacts with everyone you come in contact with and signals when you are holding onto things that aren't serving you or when you need support or inner work. Building your field increases your intuitive awareness of what is occurring in others' fields and energy systems.

This chapter will encourage you to address deeply held beliefs as you build better boundaries, heal old wounds, and process repressed emotions. Cultivating and moving energy brings up parts that resist, do not feel worthy, or require healing. This chapter will support you in working with these parts so you feel stable, sourced, and powerful.

The topics in this chapter include:

- Grounding.

- Sourcing from Earth and Divine Energies - Energy Cultivation.

- Building personal power and resiliency.

- Understanding energy centers and fields and how to maintain them.

- Healing childhood wounds.

- Building and maintaining boundaries.

- Working with the heart and repressed emotions.

- Internal protection and how not to take on others' energy.

- Deepening intuitive awareness and assessment skills.

1

FORTIFYING YOUR ENERGY BODIES

*Drawing power in and consciously working with
it is the natural progression from "I AM."*

Once you have established your "I AM," your energetic capacity will expand, and you'll become more aware of your field and its interactions with the world. Your centers and fields are fed from your central channel. The central channel gathers energy from above and below. This is called energy cultivation. You are utilizing the forces of nature and the Universe to support you with enough power and resource to do your work.

As a healer, you must source energy and draw power into your body because only a full cup should be offered to someone else. Otherwise, you risk depletion, adrenal fatigue, and the inability to handle the strength of the energy current called for in your work. You might have the potential to run a strong current, but without consistent practice, the system will be unused to it and become overwhelmed. This can lead to long-term and debilitating issues in the body and psyche.

During channeling work or healing sessions involving spirit beings like doctor spirits, angels, and guides, you request your system to function at a heightened frequency for an extended period. If you are not practiced in energetics, it can be exhausting or too challenging to attempt. Beings with significant wisdom, power, light, and love are of a higher vibration. It is your responsibility to masterfully shift frequency so it is easier on them, your client, and your body. Staying grounded and maintaining your field is crucial to receiving clear messages and guidance, and avoiding confusion and misunderstanding.

If you cannot stay grounded, you might not know when a client is overloaded or burnt out by the power coming through. You might overwork in sessions and miss important integration moments. You may have trouble being present with your clients at the end of a session in a way that will help them fully embody and allow them to go back to their lives in a healthy, grounded way. They may have never accessed this type of energy before, but if you are grounded and aware of what is happening in your field, their system will trust the energy coming through instead of sensing it as a danger and shutting down.

As you build your field, you also create a protective force to keep out the toxic energy released in healing work. Energy must go somewhere; if your field isn't strong, it can infiltrate you. Especially if you are working with people at advanced stages of illness or dealing with emotional and spiritual crises, it is imperative to have a functioning field that is constantly being replenished. The Building Your Field work gives you the energetic awareness of when you need to stop and do a quick clearing for yourself in the middle of a session or when more intensive cleansing practices are required. If you aren't doing this work, you may struggle to distinguish between your thoughts, feelings, and energy and those of others.

A bonus to building your field is that it will make you more resilient to everyday issues, including negative people, stressful situations, and the ever-increasing electrical burdens of modern technology.

Merging the Spiritual and Physical

As a divine being inhabiting a physical body, you are capable of merging the physical and spiritual realms. This means developing a heightened awareness of your physical body and sensations, your energy body and its cultivation and radiance, and the aspect of you that exists beyond these. By becoming more embodied and proficient with your energy, you can tap into the spiritual realms with greater safety and skill. Despite the benefits of embodiment and energy cultivation, you might struggle with these aspects of The Healer's Process.

You may find it challenging to be in a human body and reinforce that by saying, "It is so hard to be human, to be in a body." However, it is crucial to watch your words and consciousness. Instead, you can say, "It is fun and easy to be inside a human body. I am at home here," or even, "I am learning how to be more embodied every day."

The human experience is newer for some souls, while others have been here many times. Those who have not lived many earthly experiences might find it more challenging to be embodied in the earthly realm. These challenges can appear in worldly matters such as consistency, caring for the physical body, and relating to other humans. Sometimes, this looks like constant wonder and curiosity at mundane things such as food, smells, and communication.

Your clients may struggle with being on Earth or in their bodies. Many beings are choosing to incarnate now from other places. They come from other star systems and densities to bring a new vibration and assist in healing and the transformation of consciousness. Some are here to help with technological advances or bring new modalities and systems. Being in a messy human suit confuses those accustomed to a more refined experience. These people need guides to help them ground and express their unique energies and abilities. When you master your own embodiment and energy practices, you become a better guide.

Dissociation

You can merge the spiritual and physical by being the biological connection or conduit point (channel) between this physical, seen realm and the spiritual, unseen realms. As you master this role as a connection point or channel, you transform yourself and the collective. Dissociating from the body hinders your role as a spiritual conduit. Many people use dissociation as a coping mechanism when experiencing personal or collective trauma. Dissociating from the body serves as a form or tool of protection. Trauma, such as abuse, neglect, accidents, or severe illness, can trigger dissociation. Fear-inducing situations like war, unsafe homes, or bullying can also lead to dissociation patterns. It is prevalent in cases of sexual abuse. Dissociation is helpful because the spirit leaves the body to avoid pain and fear. However, this can make individuals feel disconnected from life, pleasure, and purpose in the long run. When stressful situations happen, they might experience a floating feeling, brain fog, and inability to focus. They might not be able to feel parts of their bodies, and life may seem overly difficult. Some freeze and dissociate when touched or during intimate moments, leading to feelings of disconnection and inability to enjoy embodied experiences. They might even engage in extreme behaviors to "feel something."

Your trauma might have been a doorway to becoming a healer. If so, it is even more essential to master embodied experience and grounding. You will more easily track dissociative clients when fully grounded and in charge of your energy field. You will notice signs such as them suddenly dropping out of the ability to communicate, the light going out in their eyes, they turn cold, or the energy you were tracking seems to go away altogether. It is a sensation you are following, so you need to be able to track physical sensations in yourself. When you notice them leaving their body, help them remain present and bring attention to the experience. Because dissociation is primarily an unconscious reaction, people need support to become aware of it. Over time, they can become more proficient at staying present even when challenging emotions or situations arise. You can help them realize that dissociation is a protection tool, but they can lead a more fulfilling life by working through underlying issues in session work. Learning about dissociation and why it might be a strategy they are leaning on puts them on the road to recovery. It offers context for their experiences and brings conscious attention to when it is happening.

When we dissociate, we can leave behind soul fragments, the basis of soul retrieval work, a shamanic practice. But all healing work brings fragmented parts of self back to the whole. Remember, we defined healing as coming back to wholeness. This includes integrating back soul parts separated from the whole when someone experiences trauma. You might practice it in a shamanic way by traveling through the realms to bring the soul part back to the body (this is a specialized training we won't explore here), or you may talk someone through a deep childhood healing, which opens the door for the soul parts to come naturally back home. Many of the healing concepts and practices of The Healer's Process focus on healing soul fragmentation and drawing together parts that have been separated from the whole. I always end energy work sessions with time focused on bringing back lost parts, as this is when a client is more capable of integrating this work. It is vital in soul retrieval work to remain grounded as it is easier to reground the soul fragments into the client's body. We work in resonance fields, and how our system operates inspires the same in others. This means that when you work with someone, your field's strength and vibration communicate with theirs, causing their field to shift to become more like yours.

Some learn how to astral travel through dissociation and leaving the body. These people are often good at lucid dreaming and dream-based healing work. Some fear that doing work to become more grounded will stop them from being able to easily travel or connect psychically. Don't worry. This isn't the case; a more solid anchor makes for safer travel.

JOURNAL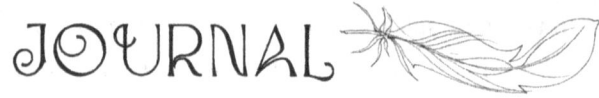

Notice:

- Can you assess feeling in every area of your body easily?

- How is your connection to your pelvis, legs, and feet?

- Does your partner remember more details of a fight, such as what you said, than you do because you have trouble remembering aspects of conflict after a resolution?

- Do you get sleepy when conflict arises and have to pass out for a while?

- Do you remember sexual experiences, or are there sections that go missing?

- Do you have consistent memories from your childhood, or are there blank periods?

Use these questions for your own illumination and also when assessing your client. Track them during sessions. Do they go cold when you touch them? Do they often fall asleep in sessions? Can they track what is going on during your work? Noticing these things will help you tune into moments of dissociation and the patterns that might appear in daily life.

Building the field requires you to fully connect to and bring energy from above and below, which we'll explore in the following sections. You might not think much of it at first, but on further exploration, you'll find this is healing in and of itself! This is because connecting to the above and below and sourcing requires you to look at your relationships with being human, being divine, trust, safety, worthiness, and even your relationships with masculine and feminine energies. You'll see where you are not fully expressing or accepting certain energies. You might also notice that you've overcompensated in one area because of an old belief that you're now ready to shift.

2

SOURCING: THE BELOW

We must root to the Earth's energy to be grounded as healers.

During my awakening, energy forcefully shot up through my body. This is common, and it is encouraged by doing "fire" practices such as Kundalini Yoga, which encourages energy to rise through the energy centers, or meditations that focus on the third eye area. As the energy rises and works through the centers, it purifies each. This helps open and awaken the gifts of each center. But, you risk becoming ungrounded and destabilized without focus and effort to become solid, comfortable, and present with the lower centers—especially the root, the energy center at the base of the pelvis, and the Lower Dantian, the energy center in the belly. My awakening destabilized me. I was too sensitive and open to participate in life fully. This lasted for years. Through the work I am guiding you through, I stabilized and fortified myself to do my sacred work and even enjoy the world without becoming overwhelmed by others. The goal of this chapter is to support you to do the same.

For many, a grounded nature is not their strong suit: all the energy flows upward, but there isn't a solid root cultivating energy from below. This can disturb the energy system and take focused effort to mend. This would be considered a "Qi (energy) Deviation." There is too much fire or upward-flowing energy and not enough water or downward-flowing energy. Your practices allow you to shift the way your energy moves consciously. Practices must feel balanced, and not all practices are helpful for everyone at every time of life. For example, suppose you are doing a lot of fire practice or experiencing spontaneous energy awakening that feels hot. In that case, you need practices to pull the energy back down, such as a water practice like qigong. Replenishing your Yin and receptive, quiet nature is essential, and grounding practices are the saving grace of overly Yang energetic overwhelm. If you have this condition, you might sweat profusely even when it isn't hot—your face may feel flushed or even break out in a rash, or your digestion might suffer. In this case, you might want to seek help from an acupuncturist or medical Qi Gong practitioner. You may need to alter your diet and take herbal formulas.

The root at the base of the pelvis and the Lower Dantian in the belly are the homes of safety, trust, belonging, and sexuality. These are common areas of trauma, and those wounds can shut down your ability to feel and draw energy into these areas. Your energy operates primarily in the lower centers at the beginning of life. Childhood or adolescence trauma can affect these centers' ability to source, hold, and radiate energy, contributing to being ungrounded. The Lower Dantian must be capable of collecting and preserving energy for successful healing. This area also gives you access to kinesthetic awareness, meaning you can track what is going on for someone else in their physical body. If these centers aren't turned on (accessible, clear, and functioning), it will be harder to feel your clients kinesthetically.

Trauma in the first center (the root at the base of the center of the pelvis) is associated with losing trust in the primary caregivers, creating mistrust of the world. Second-center (belly) issues are often related to shame of the genitals or sexual abuse. Shame experienced during potty training can shut down these areas. Many Western males are circumcised as infants, and this is a source of trauma rarely acknowledged. We'll look at practices to heal these areas in the next section.

You can become ungrounded by :

- Avoiding practices that sink awareness into your pelvis and legs and then down into the Earth or not drawing Earth energy into your body.

- Focusing primarily on opening the heart. Running only on heart energy can lead to being overly emotional, anxious, and simply feeling too much. It's important for maintaining balanced energy that focused energetic development at the front of the heart is paired with equal development of energetic awareness at the back of the heart (many people struggle with feeling energy or holding attention at the back of the heart, and it is often a place of stuck energy and emotions).

- Being very "spiritual," spending a lot of time in contemplation and communion with the higher realms, or focusing on intellect and not valuing the body's knowing can manifest as living in the head and lacking embodiment.

- Holding extrasensory gifts, astral travel, and blissing out on Spirit as higher value than being in this 'pesky human suit.'

- Prioritizing spiritual growth over practical matters can lead to difficulty navigating real-life situations. More troubling physical and mental issues can arise, including:

- Problems paying bills, getting to appointments on time, or navigating the earthly realities of life.

- Being spacey, flaky, or too "out there" and so have trouble forming relationships.

- Digestive and sexual issues.

- Difficulty "manifesting" or holding onto things.

- Energy deviations that result in ungrounded, magical thinking and even hallucinations.

- Burning out easily or adrenal issues—kidneys not supported by earth energy or cooling water energy. Too consumed by fire energy.

JOURNAL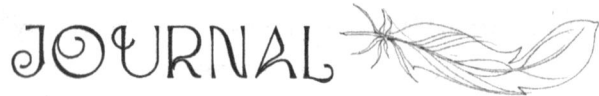

Reflect on grounding.

Which of these statements resonates with you?

- I focus on love and light. I see it as more important or powerful than the physical, mundane earthly world.

- I have a hard time:

  » paying bills

  » being punctual

  » making plans

  » taking care of my body

  » living in a body

  » with trust and safety

  » feeling my feet, legs, pelvis, sex, or belly

- I easily leave my body, dissociate, and/or travel in the astral plane.

- I focus on practices that open and activate. I am less comfortable in Yin (slow, still, and gentle) nurturing experiences, which have less value.

- I do healing and activating sessions, practices, and ceremonies but often neglect rest and integration.

- My relationship with the Earth is ...

- My relationship with my mother (or more motherly, feminine caregiver) is ...

- My relationship with my feminine is ...

- I might be blocking lower energy by:

  » disconnecting from my sexuality

  » holding shame

  » being unable to forgive my mother/ primary caregiver

The bottom line is that the most vital piece healers miss when opening their channel to healing frequencies is not being grounded within their bodies and into the Earth. Grounding must be practiced daily so you can drop quickly and easily into it. If you're not rooted and grounded when doing healing work, you risk absorbing the excess electromagnetic charges from your clients into your organs and "taking on" their emotions. When your body attempts to discharge the energy, it might shake, burp, blush, jerk, yawn, sigh, or twitch. These are not negative reactions but signal your body's desire to reach homeostasis and the need to drop in and ground more.

If ungroundedness is a problem, spend extra moments placing your attention in your pelvis and belly. Breathe into the area. Run energy from the feet up, but don't let it immediately shoot into the heart and third eye. Sink down, move slowly and sensually in the hips and pelvis, bend the knees, feel your feet, squat every day, and honor that you belong in this earth suit. Press your hands and feet upon the Earth and feel connected to this massive magnetic being below your feet. Welcome grounding actions that bring physical structure, health, dependability, and financial success. Eat grounding foods like dense root vegetables or animal products if you are open to it. Love your grounded, supported self. You can still be super-spiritual, but when you balance the core aspects of your being, you garner more power and force. Again, while many desire exploration in the upper realms and sourcing from above, focusing on grounding, safety, and trust is vital as they are the supportive base of your upper realm works.

[Practice 10: Hands and Feet]

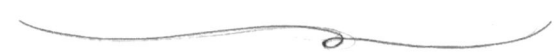

Drawing Energy from the Earth

Standing practice is the easiest way to become more grounded and cultivate Earth energy. Stand with your feet hip-distance apart or wider, toes pointing forward. Rock back and forth, feeling your feet and finding a center balance point. Let your knees become soft, and your tailbone relax downward. Soften your belly to allow breath to enter that space. You might have to jiggle your belly a bit to get the muscles to relax. Let your heart rest on your belly and feel a little space under your armpits as your shoulder blades come down and back behind you. Let your crown rise from the back center of your head so your spine elongates gently. Feel a stacking of your bones. Relax and breathe. Drop your awareness into the Earth and feel yourself below your feet. Keep working with your attention to notice as deeply into the Earth as possible, then your feet, and then your breath in your belly.

Allow energy to rise up into your body. If you can't feel this, it's ok and happening anyway. You can imagine light or elemental energy coming into your body. Keep finding an engaging posture and then relax into the stance. You may only be able to hold this briefly, but as you practice, you will improve. Be sure to shake your body, stretch out any tension you might have held, and thank the Earth.

Squatting

Squatting is the most natural resting position for human beings. In some countries, it's common to see people of all ages squatting on the ground, making food, crafting, and socializing. In the West, we are more accustomed to sitting and miss out on the benefits of a natural squat, which stretches and tones the pelvic floor. The muscles can reach their natural length and resting state in a squat and be activated when pulling energy into the body. The muscles must get full length because they are the base, the basket where our organs sit. The organs are healthy and lifted because of the expansion and contraction of the pelvic floor muscles. Squatting gives you access to full contraction but also full release. This expansion and contraction will be used to pull energy up into the body from the Earth. Squatting connects the root to the Earth, develops muscular awareness and skill, and hooks you into direct communication with the Earth, which will all help you be more grounded and allow your energy practices to have more significant effects. This is a great practice to incorporate daily as you don't have to do much more than squat down and breathe into your pelvic floor, imagining your connection to the Earth's energy rising into your body. If you can't get your heels on the ground, this is something to work toward and will be supported by stretching your calves and developing more flexibility in your ankles. Until then, you can place a rolled yoga mat or another object under your heels to help balance. Start next to a wall for support if needed. This isn't about creating pain, and if your knees, ankles, or hips hurt, take it slowly and do a little each day.

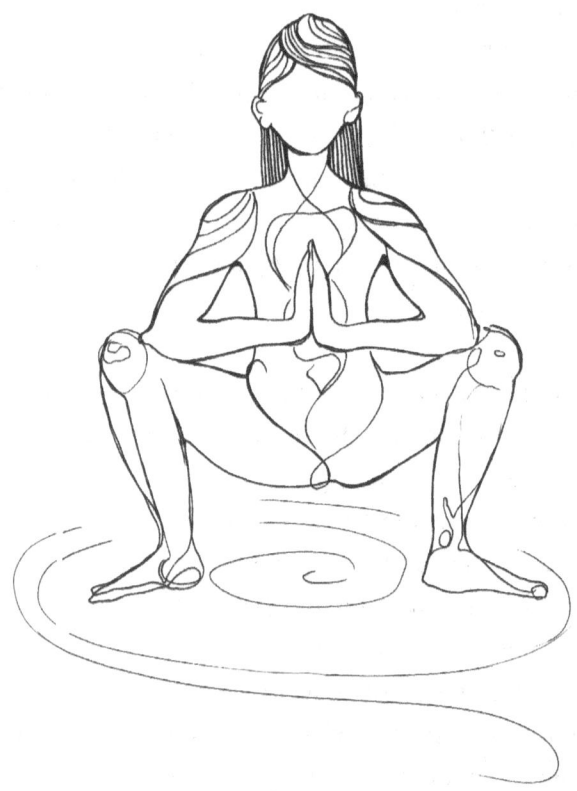

People avoid grounding and embodiment. Yet, this work inspires the greatest healing and awakening. The embodiment journey can bring up memories and emotions and feel confusing, uncomfortable, and messy. Thankfully, it also blesses us with freedom, pleasure, and expression.

[Practice 11: Squatting]

[Practice 12: Warrior Stance]

[Practice 13: Grounding into the Triple Spiral]

[Practice 14: Shaman Walk]

3

OVERCOMING SHAME AND CHILDHOOD ISSUES

Create safety, release shame, and work with your
inner child to heal your deepest wounds.

Healing shame and caregiver-related issues can help you become more grounded. Be aware that you or your clients may have addictive hyper-arousal patterns and must understand how to calm and soothe the nervous system. This means that when conditioned to anxiety, worry, stress, fear, and trauma loops, you may become, in a way, addicted to them and find comfort in these uncomfortable experiences. This hyper-arousal and hyper-vigilance can be felt as upward-flowing, jagged energy that is the opposite of connecting downward and relaxing into a trust in Earth Mother and her nurturing energy.

If you find grounding practices boring, unengaging, or unsafe, it's essential to explore why you feel this way. You may come from a chaotic, intense, or abusive home, so that environment feels "normal" to you, and grounding feels foreign. In this case, ask, "What will help me feel protected in my environment? What will help me feel safe?" It takes softness, patience, and inquiry to feel what would rewire and unwind your nervous system, so anxiety and chaos aren't your default. They might appear boring or unproductive because you don't have a solid relationship with calmness and peace. They might even be scary. We can create all sorts of situations to prove our lack of safety and trust so that the neurological pathways continue to wear the old familiar groove of anxiety and fear.

Your mind can tell you you are safe, but you will still feel fear and anxiety if your nervous system isn't experiencing that. Movement and energy practices help your nervous system heal as you work with your consciousness to uncover your beliefs about yourself and the world. Over time, you increase the capacity of the nervous system to feel calm and safe.

Learning to Reconnect

Shame stops connection; it keeps us from feeling like we deserve to pull energy into our bodies. It is a negative self-evaluation that anchors that there is something wrong with you as a person. In your practice, ask to open and release shame from your body and life. People often hold shame in the womb space (lower abdomen in any person). In Daoist tradition, we hold shame alongside grief and sadness in the lungs. The lungs are linked to the large intestine, so the belly is again connected to this energy. Tuning into shame can trigger grief and sadness, and you may need a good cry. The other energies of the lungs are confidence, integrity, and honor. So, when you ask for shame to be released, you can request to be filled with these beneficial energies. So often, when shame was instilled, confidence diminished.

[Practice 15: Releasing Shame]

JOURNAL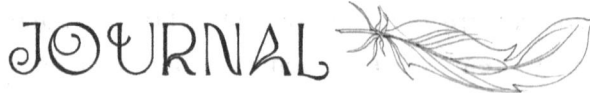

- Around what do I feel shame?

- What was I shamed for as a child?

- Was I shamed for something in a past relationship?

- Where would I like to see myself express more confidence? What is one thing I could begin today to express myself more?

Earth Our Mother

Often, the source of our shame, along with a whole host of beliefs, comes from our mother or primary care provider when we were children. For this reason, the word "mother" and connecting to the Great Mother beneath our feet may not feel safe. The best place to resolve mother issues is by forming a deep personal relationship with Mother Earth. Connecting with your mother may be difficult, but loving, respecting, and honoring the Earth is easy. Over time, this can help heal your energetic and emotional wounds from your actual mother. Simply being with Earth Mother, resting in her wild places, speaking directly to her, and devotionally connecting through gardening and land restoration can open deep healing. You will develop a healthy, nurturing relationship and transmute your feelings of disconnection and pain.

[Practice 16: Healing Through Mother Earth]

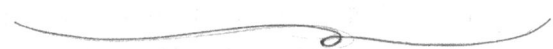

Inner Child Work

When you connect to nurturing energies from below and above, childhood wounds may arise. Many shut down abilities and openness in childhood. Maybe you were scared by what you saw, heard, or experienced psychically. Perhaps you were punished for sharing things that you saw or knew. As you reopen these abilities, you may feel confronted by old feelings of shame, fear, and doubt and hear a judgmental voice installed in your consciousness by these experiences. You may even feel a deep sense of being unsafe. These arising sensations, thoughts, and feelings may require inner child work, as so many issues do.

This will look like meeting, speaking to, and listening to your inner child and integrating their wisdom and energy back into your body. This isn't a one-and-done situation because you are forming relationship with these early parts of self from different times in your childhood. You may need to sit with and pour love and understanding into a child part for some time. Just as with any child, patience is key.

Through this process, you may uncover trauma or new information, and seeking support from a counselor or healer is helpful. Sometimes, aspects of childhood were closed off because you couldn't handle them at the time. If something presents itself, know you have the stability and tools to address it. This doesn't mean you need to do this alone, and a specialist can help you get through this more easily.

[Practice 17: Inner Child]

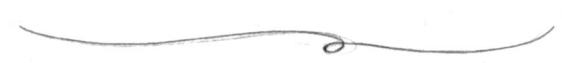

Healing Parental Wounds

Claiming your magic is a deep process of uncovering your wounds, clearing energy, emotions, and beliefs of the past, and stepping into greater understanding of your experiences. Healers often have specific wounds regarding gifts and abilities. You are working through layers of liberation to feel more free and capable of tapping into your intrinsic talents and passions.

All people have childhood wounds, and as a healer, you will witness these wounds as you help others process their past. Doing your inner work and confronting your past enables you to understand how to guide and support others.

[Practice 18: Letter to Heal Childhood Wounds]

When you see the pains in your body and heart as opportunities for growth instead of something to hide from, you allow deep healing to occur and your true nature of love to emerge.

Don't expect these changes to happen overnight. Further opportunities to make decisions that feed old patterns will arise repeatedly. The intensity of desire and wanting to meet your needs can be doorways for previous ways to emerge. Come back to your body, your breath, and self-love, and gently ask what you need to feel calm and supported, and then take those steps and make those requests of your friends, family, partners, home, and guides. This will help shift long-standing addiction to intensity and anxiety.

From this place, you can cultivate peace and presence, opening up your personal practices to be even more supportive and regenerative. In unfamiliarity with a new way of being, your ego will try to break down this calming and nurturing new pattern and reinstate old ways. Recognizing your past and its effect on how your nervous system responds to situations and having compassion and gentleness can help unwind these tendencies to return to old patterns. It isn't always in the intense and exciting breakthroughs that the work happens. It might be in the most subtle noticing you have ever done.

4

SOURCING: THE ABOVE

When fully grounded and rooted in Earth Mother,
you can rise far beyond your imaginings.

You are meant to receive Divine Light from above, which then radiates throughout your being. Although we are all a part of the Divine, we can sometimes disconnect ourselves from Source frequency and prevent it from entering our fields. By becoming aware of how you shut down and learning how to consciously open yourself up to the above, you will become more radiant and connected to the teachings of the higher guides and Divine wisdom.

JOURNAL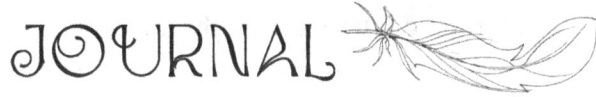

Do you relate to the following:

- I focus on the mundane, working and getting things accomplished.

- I am sluggish and swing more toward depression.

- I have a hard time:

  - » Seeing the bright side.

  - » Receiving messages

  - » Feeling connected to the All That There Is, Light, Guidance, Source, or God.

- My relationship with my father (or more masculine caregiver) and the masculine is ...

- My relationship with God is ...

- I might be blocking upper frequencies by ...

  - » Eating heavy and processed foods.

  - » Shutting down my special gifts, magical abilities, messages, and visions.

  - » Being afraid of what I might see, hear, or experience if I let myself be fully open.

While some perceive a correlation between father/mother or masculine/feminine and their relationship to celestial/terrestrial frequencies, others will not. It might even feel backward. I divide these opposing forces to examine the root causes of wounds, beliefs, or stagnant energies and see if correlations support your process. You might not resonate with binary categorization or see masculine and feminine through this lens. I am offering these as reflection points for your illumination. The opportunity is to explore all aspects of yourself fully, do the deeper work, and allow yourself access to as much information, light, love, and energy as possible.

Connecting to the Universal Flow

You move through life differently when you align with the universal energy flow. You realize you always have access to this unending stream of energy. The above is light. You can begin your journey by holding your arms up and imagining gathering light into your body. Draw your arms down and see yourself transforming into light; it fills your being and becomes a part of every cell of your body. You are once again forming a relationship. This time, it is with the Divine and the light of above. This might require addressing your beliefs about your worthiness to receive this kind of light, information, and power.

[Practice 19: Connecting to the Above Via Your Star Cord]

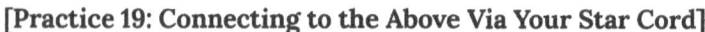
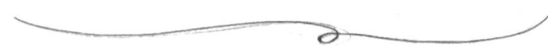

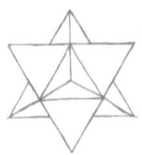

HELD

Held

In energetic balance,

Between

Divine Father and Earth Mother

Above and below.

Receiving and giving

Giving and receiving.

I own my path upon this Earth guided by the Light.

Illuminate my darkest places, my deepest
wounds, and my forgotten shadows.

Ease overcomes me as I surrender.

I am open to containing that which is my birthright.

The above,

The below,

The left,

The right,

The front,

The back,

The internal,

The external,

The balance allows me to see everything I know
until I know again. I am remembered.

I am shattered open and brought back together.

Held in knowledge and love.

Gratitude washes through my being.

Thank you, Mother.

Thank you, Father.

I am held

5

THE AURIC FIELD AND ENERGY CENTERS

You were never just a body. You have always been so much more.

Energy fields flow through and surround your body like all living things. Even things you might not consider living have fields. These fields are a protective cocoon that constantly reflects health and well-being and interacts with all other fields in the area. It is a warning system, a filter, and a source of information. It is through these fields that you interact with the world. You take in information, emotions, and either toxic or healing energy through these fields. They must be addressed in healing for lasting results.

The concept of the auric field has been a topic of discussion throughout history in various cultures, both ancient and modern. Many acknowledge a seven-layer auric field, corresponding to seven main energy centers. Others describe more or fewer primary fields flowing around and through the body. In this section, we'll explore three primary fields as known in Medical Qi Gong, which connect to the three Dantians (belly, heart, and mind energy centers) as it can be confusing to describe more fields when, for most of us, we won't have a tangible experience of many fields until we have been doing this work for quite some time. Over time and with practice, you will learn to differentiate and work with the different layers, experiencing them as you are intuitively guided. I will also use the terms field and auric field to mean the full expression of all the fields together.

Radiating out from the central channel, energy centers, organs, and tissues, your field uniquely expresses how you are physically, emotionally, spiritually, and energetically. Before an illness manifests, it is embedded in the field. This is important because treating the field and removing toxic energy can keep the body from later manifesting disease. When a tumor is removed, it may reappear if there are no energetic clearings of the fields, along with addressing associated emotional stagnations. When we see, feel, or sense the areas of the field holding toxic energy and support its removal, we help relieve the body's overall toxic burden. This has a healing effect on all levels of being.

What Damages the Auric Field?

Both internal and external factors can invade and damage the auric field. From your inner state, you damage your fields with suppressed emotions. Please notice I am saying suppressed emotions, not emotions. People get the idea that being spiritual means they should never have what they consider negative emotions. Having emotions isn't harmful; they are a normal part of being human. Repression and stuffing down emotions cause issues. This doesn't mean cruelty, callousness, or overreacting is called for. These aren't healthy expressions because they may harm others or create toxic behavior patterns, disconnecting you from peace.

You want to be able to feel, acknowledge, and find healthy expression of your feelings. Feelings are not who or what you are; they are like passing clouds bringing important information. When you over-identify with them, they embed more deeply in your system, meaning that instead of being with and moving the feeling's energy, you might identify with it and create a structure around it linked to your identity. This shuts down the natural flow of energy and creates blockages. Many people tend to avoid fully experiencing their emotions. Fear of the emotion is often more intense than facing it.

When one experiences trauma, one tends to internalize that trauma and hold onto it, and harmful emotional residues radiate out into the fields. You can damage your fields by holding onto resentment, anger, and rage instead of cultivating forgiveness for yourself and others. What one puts out, they get back. Negative thought forms directed at others will eventually come home. Repetitive negativity and negative self-talk deplete the fields.

Damage can occur from external factors such as adverse environmental influences, physical traumas, or energy you bring into your field from others. Lack of sleep, poor diet, and addictions weaken the fields.

This doesn't mean you are stuck with a "damaged field." You can shift and heal issues in the fields. They are constantly being regenerated based on what you resonate with and can be consciously cleaned and strengthened. This is done through cultivating heightened awareness, energy, and movement practices, moving stuck emotions that have become toxic, building energy in the central channel and energy centers, prayer, meditation, and positive thoughts and deeds.

The next chapter will teach you more about cleansing and purifying your fields.

The Three Dantians

The three primary protective fields are connected to the three Dantians, or primary energy centers in the body. Working with these three centers builds and supports your auric field. In Chapter 1, you began your work by focusing on the central channel, which helps build your field. The Lower Dantian (belly energy center) feeds and nurtures the first protective layer of your field. This layer, just outside the physical body, about an inch or more, is the last layer of defense before something invades the body, and it is connected to the immune system. It holds the codes of the physical form. You can see how important it is to connect to the belly center and cultivate energy reserves there.

The second field corresponds with the middle Dantian (heart energy center). You strengthen this field by focusing on the heart, cultivating and radiating love, compassion, and inner peace. This field extends a foot or more from the body. Because it is connected to the heart and emotions, this field radiates the colors and lights seen in auric photography. If you can read auras and see colors in people's fields, this is usually the one you read. Emotions strongly affect the field, which creates changes in colors.

Here are the subtle energies of the organs and repressed emotions. This field interprets emotions and feelings from others, so it is the field of empathy and helps us to navigate social experiences. It protects us from negativity and criticism and can be damaged in childhood by growing up in a highly negative or critical home. When tuning into this field, you can become aware of stuck and repressed emotional energies and help move them. This can create an opening for emotional catharsis and movement from density to lightness. If this field isn't cleared, toxic emotional residue will eventually settle into the first field and then deeper and deeper into the body, creating disease in the physical form.

The third field corresponds to the Upper Dantian (mind energy center). It flows from a few feet to several hundred yards from the central channel. This is dependent on spiritual growth and development. You may recognize the strength of this field in spiritually advanced teachers you have met. They can fill an entire room with their presence. This field is associated with your intuitive awareness, inspiration, and spiritual insight. Tuned to the spiritual body, this field interacts with the world from a spiritual level and draws others on the same spiritual path.

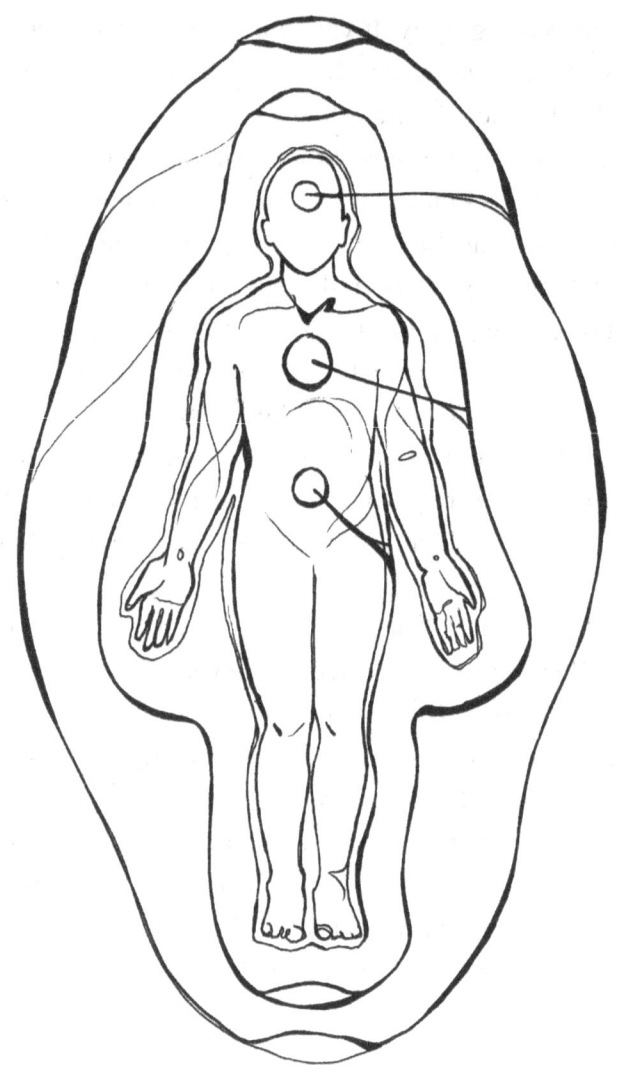

Diagnosing the Fields

You don't have to see the fields to become aware of them. You might experience colors or densities or have a more kinesthetic feeling or a knowing about the fields. Trust your insights and awareness, and over time, they will develop. Start by tuning into your field regularly. Sit in meditation and sense it with all of your capabilities. Notice anything you can. A clear and strong field will feel light and radiating.

It might have lovely colors, and the vibration feels good. Issues may show up as dense, heavy spots, sensations of holes, darkness, stickiness, or a tar-like substance. You might even sense objects, ropes, and cords to and from others. In general, the brighter the field, the healthier it is. Notice areas that are easy to connect to and where you have more trouble.

A dark, black, grey, and dull field isn't healthy and could signal disease already in the body, even if symptoms haven't manifested. You might be able to feel more with your hands. Use your hands to feel all along the field so that even if you can see, you will get feedback on what the hands and other senses communicate. You might feel sliminess, stickiness, a sludge-like sensation, or sense a hole or dense area that can be hot or cold. You will discover over time what these different messages mean to you.

Once you become good at tuning into the fields, you will recognize how the information corresponds to areas or organs of the body. By clearing the densities and sludge-like energy from the fields, you support healing in the tissues and organs.

Even if you are doing physical, structural bodywork, checking and clearing the fields is essential. This is because of the interconnected nature of the various bodies. Going directly into the body can cause the energy from the field to infiltrate the area. Clearing first helps the tissues adjust and release tension without the next wave of toxic energy flowing directly into the area. By working from outward to inward, you have a better degree of success. After working in the physical body, it is wise to revisit the field, recheck it, clear it as needed, and patch it up with light from the Divine.

[Practice 20: Assess and Clear Your Field]

[Practice 21: Assessing Another's Field]

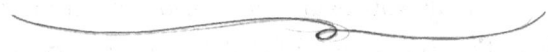

6

BOUNDARIES

Boundaries are clarity in action.

We can't talk about building the field without mentioning boundaries because weak boundaries create weaknesses in the energy field, and a weak energy body creates conditions for poor boundaries to emerge. One feeds the other back and forth. It is vital to address weaknesses and wounds in your energy field while cultivating better boundaries so that you are not vulnerable to attack and being drained.

Boundaries define us, yet they're often faulty because we're not taught how to recognize them or what they feel like in childhood. We might have had no boundaries or been so railroaded that we don't understand healthy ones. Being brought up in a home with a lot of criticism, fighting, or abuse, or not being allowed to say no to an adult or express wants and needs can mean we need to learn boundaries as adults. Add in an education environment where boundaries are overrun by administration and peers, and all sorts of issues emerge.

Many people who identify as empaths were brought up in unstable homes. You are safer if you can track and feel what is happening at home. If you can read the first signs of negative emotions, you can escape a situation that may cause pain or harm. Better still, learn how to process toxic energy, and you might help diffuse nasty situations. Like many things we learn as children to keep us safe, these skills can harm us as adults. You may approach the world with a very open, porous field—constantly processing others' energy and trying to harmonize situations. This is exhausting and, in the long term, weakens health and life-force. The good news is that you can learn to use your hard-earned empath skills in your work for the benefit of your clients without taking on too much and feeling responsible for processing everything. This is done by understanding your energy system and its way of engaging with the world, clearing and fortifying it, and building better boundaries.

Outer World and Inner World Boundaries

With boundaries, there are psychological, energetic, and physical components. If you go to a therapist, they might help you with boundaries by encouraging you to state your needs and wants and supporting you to say no more often. However, you need to learn what you want and how to communicate it alongside energy practices to purify, build, and maintain the boundary system, which is the body's auric field. As you work on your energetic boundaries, your ability to say no and honor yourself and others will naturally improve. By working on your physical, real-world boundaries, your energy fields strengthen.

Life changes as you build these energetic boundaries and become more aware of your auric field. You stop accepting abuse or being taken advantage of and create better boundaries over time. Resentment fades as it stems from chronically poor boundaries. You may even confront how you might manipulate or railroad others, disrespecting their boundaries. That isn't a successful strategy for maintaining healthy relationships, but it is often done when unconscious of habits and patterns.

As you uncover your patterns and make changes, you discover life is a constant evolution. You might realize you have maintained relationships that don't serve that evolution. Even though every relationship has the potential to teach you about yourself and inspire growth, they are not all meant to last forever. Relationships that don't evolve, grow, or change as you evolve become more challenging to maintain. As you become curious about the infinite, you want to go deeper in all directions: in love, friendships, business partnerships, and with your family.

Realizing you're in a relationship based on an old program that is no longer true shifts everything. The relationship will only survive if the other person is curious or if a lot of work is done to maintain the dynamic. Sometimes, when you set boundaries, people who are used to your previous behavior may resist. They may use old tactics to manipulate you into acting differently. Others will respond positively and begin to trust and respect you more. Often, people fight back for a bit. They test. They try different things. They might get upset at how unfair you are being. Eventually, people will understand and appreciate your boundaries. They will learn to respect them if they value their relationship with you.

For many years, I struggled with boundaries. I had trouble differentiating my emotions from those I picked up from others. I often felt confused when deciding what I wanted or liked. I merged easily with others, shifting myself so they would feel good. Learning about my energy body and how to process and feel my emotions healthily, I began enforcing stronger boundaries in my relationships. I have learned to love myself more and change my behaviors to reflect not where I came from but the person I desire to be. Sometimes, I am still uncomfortable when my needs don't align with someone I love. Moving past any judgment, shame, or fear arising from advocating for my needs is a practice. It is also a practice to speak up and have tough conversations without experiencing emotional overwhelm.

Suppose you are at an event where people go through healing processes, such as a retreat, workshop, or ceremony. In that case, you must be even more grounded and sourced so your energetic field and boundaries are stronger to avoid confusing their experience with your own. If you are more contained within yourself, you can do the work you came for and not just manage the group's energy. As a healer, you must master your ability to merge and separate from others. It is helpful to be open to others' energy to read and affect it, but it is also important to detach and close the connection so that you are not left drained or taking on the caretaker role.

Let us further break down different aspects of boundaries so you can assess where you are with each type and initiate changes as needed.

Physical Boundaries

Physical boundaries can be all things in the physical environment that affect you. This is time, place, and physical safety and well-being. You might see a lack of physical boundaries show up in:

- Saying no.

- Honoring your office or working hours.

- Tracking and managing time in sessions.

- Being clear at the beginning of consultations or sales calls of the structure of the call and the time you have scheduled for it (and sticking to it).

- Taking days off work and social media.

- Accepting inappropriate behavior in sessions, such as sexual suggestiveness, lateness, or constant rescheduling.

- Issues arising from working with friends and family.

JOURNAL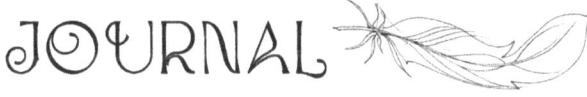

Look for patterns in boundary issues when they appear in your session work. See the list above. What does this say about you? What do you want to change? What would you have access to if you changed these things, and how would life change?

Emotional Boundaries

These are issues that affect your emotional state and well-being. What are you tolerating? Healthy emotional boundaries require determining what feels good and is desirable and what doesn't, acknowledging what is true for you, advocating for yourself, and stating what you will and will not accept in your relationships. The easiest way to be pulled away from spiritual development is to be emotionally drained by your relationships. You might see a lack of emotional boundaries in:

- Trying to process all the emotions in a relationship where the other person is sullen and shut down. (Doing all the emotional labor)

- Taking on others' feelings as your own.

- Accepting emotional abuse and manipulation.

JOURNAL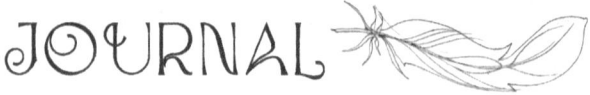

Look again for patterns. See the list above. What do you want to change? What would you have access to if you changed these things, and how would life change?

Spiritual Boundaries

Here, we look at your boundaries in relationships with spirits and guides. We'll explore this topic more fully in The Sacred Container and The Work, but in summary, lack of spiritual boundaries might show up in:

- Lacking clarity on spiritual working hours and what you are available for.

- Not being clear in your requests.

- Accepting constant interruptions, especially if they are affecting sleep.

- Over-channeling and burnout.

JOURNAL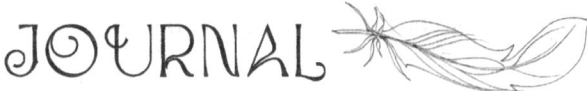

Look again for patterns. See the list above. What do you want to change? What would you have access to if you changed these things, and how would life change?

Energetic Boundaries

These boundaries concern your energy, energy body, and internal energy reserves. Because these feel less concrete than physical or emotional boundaries, which often can be associated with feeling states and sensations, you need to be more aware of these boundaries. You may have been trained in your early life to constantly merge energetically with others and absorb their energy in the same way that people absorb emotions from others. You can also consider, in this category, your vital life force, which keeps you going, and the tendency to exert yourself past your internal reserves, leading to constant exhaustion.

Lack of energetic boundaries may present as:

- Feeling responsible for another's energy.

- Trying to transmute everything in your own system.

- Taking on others' pain in an attempt to help them.

- Not doing regular clearing and healing work for yourself.

- Working on people without their consent.

- Exhausting your energetic reserves often especially in service to others.

JOURNAL

Look again for patterns. See the list above. What do you want to change? What would you have access to if you changed these things, and how would life change?

In all of these categories, you can also be the one pushing against or not honoring boundaries.

JOURNAL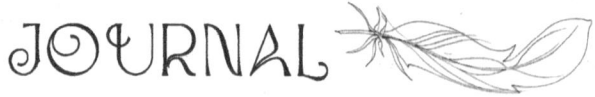

Which of these do you resonate with? Use the above categories to dive deeper into possible boundary issues, reflecting on where you learned this and what it might take to shift this old pattern.

- I let people run over me.

- At the end of a session or a day, I often feel sick, drained, incapacitated, stressed, or emotional.

- I carry people with me and think about them a lot.

- I have a hard time saying NO.

- I let people talk me into things.

- I energetically work on people I don't know when I go out in public.

- People often try to take advantage of me.

- Sometimes I can't tell where I stop, and others begin.

- I push people around and talk them into things or don't notice when I am not honoring others' boundaries.

- I have trauma that might have broken my field.

- I engage in relationships in which I morph into the other person.

- My self-care goes out of the window when I am in a relationship.

- I can ask, "Does this serve my highest and best?", get an internal answer, and follow its guidance.

- I have great boundaries. People know where I stand.

7

SHIELDING

Radiance is its own protection.

ften, boundaries are taught with an emphasis on putting up a big shiny shield to live in to protect you from the world. This can work well for some people, but as healers, we want to feel and engage in the world intimately. A big scary shield may keep out the information and energy we need to access and work with. It might even keep clients away entirely.

So, while building your auric field, you only actively put up an opaque shield if absolutely required. Know that a robust system sourced from the Earth and the Divine will keep you safe. You can benefit from visualizing your field because where you place your attention, energy flows and strengthens. If you want to imagine and infuse colors into your field, gold and pink are effective colors that are easy for others to engage with because they don't reflect too much back at the person. A shiny silver field, for example, can be too reflective, causing the person's pain and emotional turmoil to mirror back at them. This might be helpful in some situations, but in the healing room, it isn't going to serve you or your client.

Shielding is a common practice because people fear feeling and coming in contact with "toxic" people and emotions. There is no reason to fear people or emotions (unless you are in danger). Your work in this book will build a robust field and a vital internal environment. In most cases, there is no need for further protection. You will learn further spiritual protection considerations later.

Connecting to the Heart

As you build your field, the heart will play a substantial role. The heart has 5,000 times the brain's electromagnetic power and creates the body's largest electromagnetic field. The heart is constantly interacting with the environment through its toroidal energy field. The energy is scooping outward and then coming back to itself. It constantly picks up information and relays it to the brain and the rest of the body.

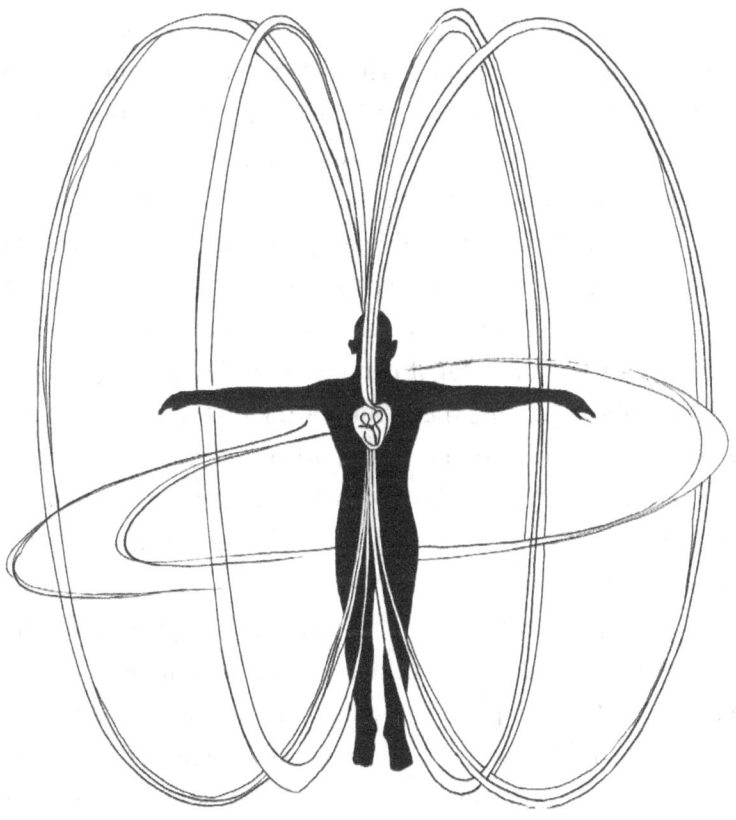

The heart is the home of the Middle Dantian, which houses your emotions, empathy, and ability to be aware of and communicate about emotions in others. Here, you track others' emotional experiences and read past emotions affecting your clients. The heart is the secret key to your intuition. You may think intuition lies in the upper center, but the heart is the true guide and holds the key to discernment. When you focus on this area, communication with your higher self emerges naturally. The heart tracks, receives, and sends information regarding emotions. It is easily shut down by focusing too much on the rational mind and can also be closed through abuse, trauma, and shock.

The heart processes and stores your emotions. Acknowledging, feeling, and moving your emotions helps you have a clear, open heart. Anything that shuts down the heart influences your ability to authentically perceive and assess your clients and the world around you. The heart wants clarity, openness, and alignment with a virtuous life. When the heart is aligned, it radiates inner peace and joy. When it isn't, it is flooded with anxiety or manic unrest.

Focusing your attention on the heart, clearing old emotions, and building its vitality through cultivating the virtues of inner peace and gratitude strengthens and expands the heart field. This, in turn, strengthens and expands your second protective field. When the heart field is strong and vital, it can more easily interact with others and their emotions, feeling them but not taking them on as your own.

The heart is also connected to the voice and the breath. Singing, toning, mantra, and breath work open and cleanse the heart. The sound of the heart is "Ha." Use a high to low inflecting tone, "Ha," to release stuck emotions in the heart, field, and body. Toning the sound from low to high cultivates joy. Smiling and laughter (ha, ha, ha!) soothe the heart, as do connection and touch from another person or animal. Gentle sighing helps the heart relax and rest. A loving and caring attitude opens the heart. At times, after experiencing pain, you may need to make a conscious effort to cultivate love and compassion. This means initiating loving care toward ourselves and others while being open to forgiving ourselves, our experiences, others involved, God or Source, and even places. Through this, we set the heart free.

[Practice 22: Focus on the Heart]

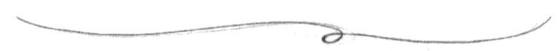

8

REPRESSED EMOTIONS
AND CATHARSIS

The poisons in the well are our repressed emotions.

You might notice a strong theme in The Healer's Process: recognizing and opening to what has been hidden. All too often, we repress our true selves, abilities, and, most of all, our emotions because it doesn't feel safe to be authentic and real in our homes, schools, or communities. Over time, we take on more and more beliefs and views that are not our truth but become so ingrained that we mistake them for our own.

Those called to the healer's path are sensitive, as it is an important part of the calling. It will serve you and help your clients. You have to be sensitive to feel what others are feeling and guide them to a new way of being in the world. You have to be sensitive to connect to energy and spirit. This sensitivity, this gift, is often seen as a curse, and many of us have spent our whole lives being called oversensitive, a crybaby, or worse. We have been shamed repeatedly for doing what we do: feel. To manage in this society, we learn useful skills. They are the skills of repressing, stuffing down, judging, dismissing, medicating, and hating our emotions. What is wrong in this situation isn't us but the larger system. We have learned that emotions are bad, messy, inconvenient, shameful, and disgusting. They don't get us ahead in the logical world, so they must be controlled, managed, and hidden.

As we shut down, we clutter our inner space, body, and field with toxic, old, repressed energies. They overfill us, and as we repress their existence, we lose connection to our truth. Emotions are valuable. Just as they are. When they are allowed, appreciated, and can run their natural course, they simply exist. They happen, we feel them, we healthily express them, and they give us feedback about our environment, boundaries, and what is acceptable and what isn't. They inspire our creativity and passion for serving. Our emotions are the glue that keeps our families and friendships together, and they are signals when we need to make changes in those relationships.

Being a healer is about being authentic and open. We are designed to feel, recognize, accept, and deal with every emotion. The process of coming back to full acceptance and expression can be intense. The more you have stored, judged, and shamed, the more must be moved, felt, and processed. Sometimes, you may feel like you're going through a complete breakdown. These are also breakthroughs. When I stopped taking psychotropic medications, I spent a lot of time crying. Not a few tears here and there, but hours of uncontrollable weeping. I have seen this in others who have gone off medications for depression and anxiety, those healing from addiction, and those who had to repress emotions to survive. This turns out to be almost everyone.

Suddenly, everything that was not felt comes rushing back to be experienced and moved. This is often when people judge and demonize the emotions or tears and seek to fix them by finding ways to shut them down. This might look like a range of coping mechanisms, addictions, and distractions. We have pathologized emotions so much that simply having them makes us feel broken and wrong. Many people you work with will be at painful odds with themselves as you guide them to feel and release emotions as they have felt unsafe and inexperienced in this process.

The more stuck energy and emotions, the more it requires moving energy. To shift these repressed energies, doing active meditations that move the body and incorporate strong movements, breath, and sound is helpful. This dynamic approach gives us access to releasing old, stuck energies. It helps quiet the mind and relax the body by moving the stickiness and repression. There are specific modalities for this, such as OSHO Dynamic Mediation or 5 Rhythms Dance. These are structured modalities that mix intensity and stillness. You can create your own form by picking several music tracks. Begin by connecting to your body and breath with gentle movement, work up to a faster, ecstatic dance, make sounds, shake, and let yourself go, and then come back to stillness at the end. You can use the techniques in this book to connect to the breath, sound, and cleansing and purification processes, as discussed in the next section. This can be a highly cathartic experience that creates powerful shifts. You might have to move through judgment of the practice itself. It can feel silly to jump around your living room or shake, moan, and cry while you flop on the floor. Notice that you were taught to feel this way about something intrinsically human.

When cultivated as a practice, this is a valuable tool for moving energy. There will always be new emotions to process, experiences to move through, and energies that must be released so that clarity can once again be found.

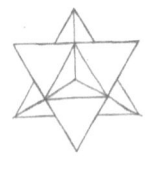

THE VESSEL

I am a vessel.

I am full, pure, holding light.

It is up to me what I bring in and what I release.

I am willing to spill out all that does not serve my highest expression.

I come home to holding,

Collecting,

Intentional in all actions.

I release, and I gather like the infinitely shifting clouds.

I am satisfied to squeeze out every drop.

And then converge in a new creative force that
will soothe and nourish the parched land.

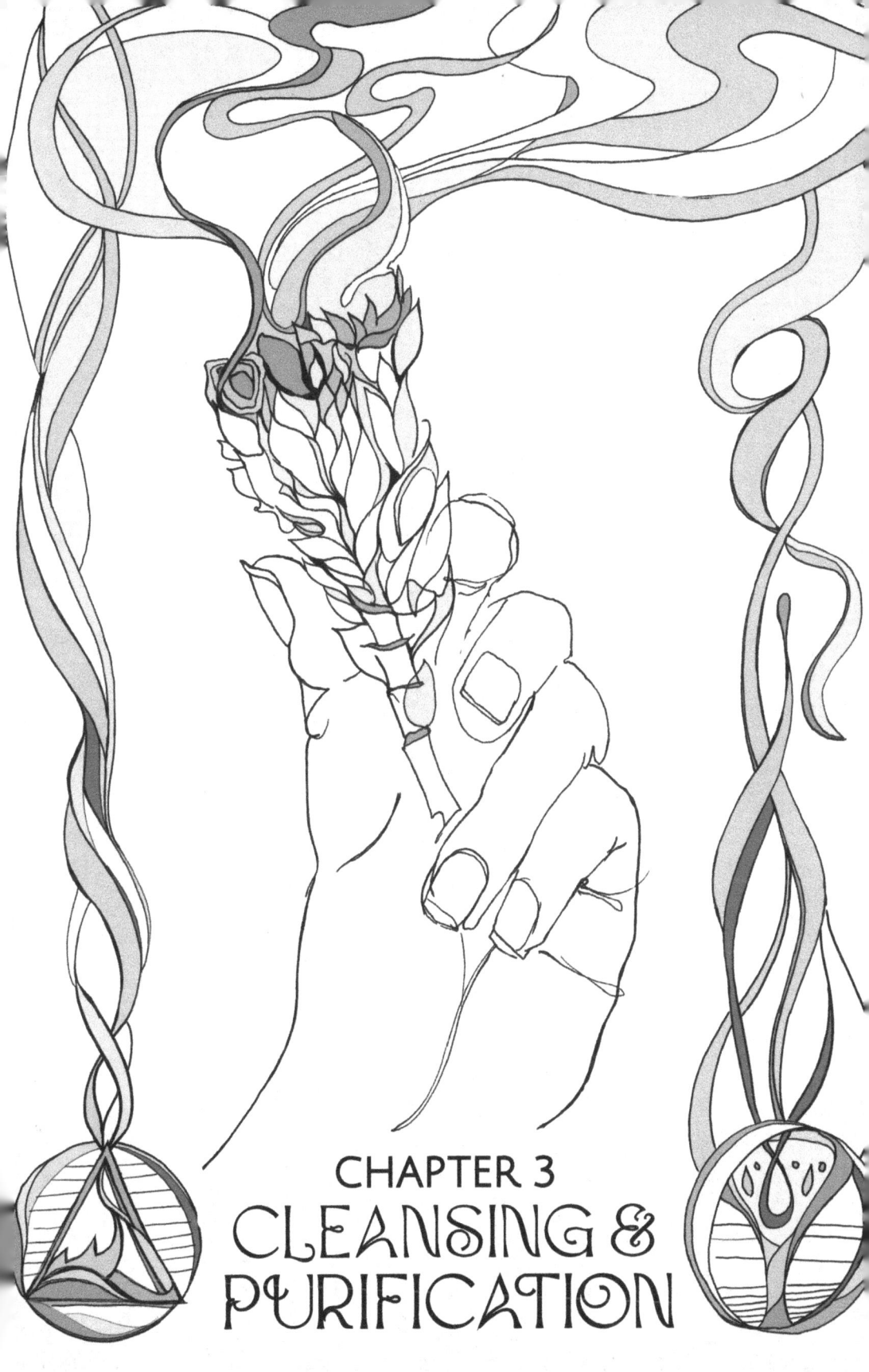

CHAPTER 3
CLEANSING & PURIFICATION

CLEANSING AND PURIFICATION

T his chapter illuminates the foundational tools of all healing work. No matter your modality, you will clear away what isn't serving and bring in the new. Despite being prime healing aspects, practitioners often overlook or misunderstand them. However, you will understand what to do with the energy stirred up in sessions and life. You will feel clear, radiant, and safe from absorbing energy from your clients. Your healing space, home, and life will radically upgrade and shift by using these tools and understanding these concepts.

This chapter builds on the last two because you must have the basics of energetic anatomy and the ability to assess issues in the field and body. This chapter helps you understand what to do next with what you sense. You will take the practices you have been doing to the next level and develop an understanding of how these concepts fit into a healing session.

The topics in this chapter include:

- Why cleansing and purification are the cornerstones of all healing work.

- Developing clarity and discernment.

- Developing effective strategies for cleansing and purifying self, clients, spaces, and tools.

- How to stop taking on energy from others.

- How to work with toxic energy released in sessions so it doesn't affect you.

- Feeling clearer, less bogged down, and safe even when you have a lot of clients.

1

PROTECTING YOUR ENERGY

*Cleansing and purification are the
cornerstones of all healing work.*

Y ou have gone from the central channel of the "I AM" and
expanded into the field around the body, and now are
interacting with the next level outward. You are shifting from
an internal focus to recognizing and interacting with what isn't you.
You will become present with the subtle shifts that need to happen to
open up deep healing and create the space for illumination to enter.

In this section, I'll cover cleansing and purification concepts and
techniques for you, your clients, and your healing and home spaces.
It can be detrimental to your physical, spiritual, emotional, and
mental health and well-being if you aren't utilizing cleansing and
purification regularly.

When I first started, I believed that at the core of everything,
we are all one, all is light, and I was fully protected from taking
anything on from others. It is a beautiful belief and has served me
well. Still, I have learned from years of practice and study that those
who incorporate cleansing and purification are healthier, clearer,
and more effective. I've also met shamans and healers who do very
little of this work. They clear others but not themselves. After many
years, the consequence can be a disease or issue in the body or life.

Cleansing and purifying practices were less necessary when we
lived closer to nature and bathed in springs, rivers, and oceans,
burned fires in our homes, and had our bare feet on the Earth—which
are all naturally detoxifying. We didn't live in such high-density,
stressful environments. Nevertheless, teachings from ancient

lineages spoke of how to cleanse and purify with the elements and specific meditations. Regular, intense cleansing practices of sweating and fasting were standard for healers. They were in tune with the land and used herbs and stones to support them. People living more traditional lives still engage in these practices. In our modern world of emotional and spiritual baggage and toxic energy, I recommend taking these practices seriously for your sake and for all you come into contact with.

Most people are gummed up in their fields and bodies. Our physical and energetic toxic load is staggering. I do a lot of work in this area because getting people to a base level of functioning without outside energy holding them down is vital. It is tough to connect to mission, purpose, and joy or to have a successful relationship under the burden of so much accumulated sludge. People often have no concept of moving energy and emotions through their systems and little ability to draw in new light, love, and power. This density makes awakening and knowing themselves that much harder. As healers and guides, I believe we are here to help people figure out how to live inside a human body at this moment of significant change. That starts with us, our space, and how we model energetics for others.

I am often asked, "How do I keep from taking on others' energy?" I've met incredible practitioners so loaded with other people's energy that they can hardly see straight. As discussed, it starts with coming home to yourself, nurturing the field through grounding and sourcing, and building healthy boundaries. The next phase is to understand cleansing and purification.

When to Use Cleansing and Purifying Practices

Cleansing and purification are done before, during, and after session work. These techniques will keep residual energetics from attaching to you, taking up residence in your space, or affecting your next client. As beliefs, emotional blocks, and trauma are released, so too is energy. The more aware you are of this and how to work with it, the less likely it is to lodge again in your client's field, attach to you, or hang around waiting for the most vulnerable person to show up.

Taking on too much from others happens for many reasons. Some people's systems are more naturally open and receptive than others. Even during online, phone work, talk therapy, or doing readings, people release energy and trauma, their emotional body is activated, and things are moving. Out in the world, very few people understand what their energy is doing and are spewing emotions, energy, and thought forms all over the place. The Daoists call this "Pernicious Qi." Energy has to go somewhere; you are in charge of where it goes in session work. It can also be a bit sneaky, so cleaning up thoroughly is always a good idea.

Awareness of intense energy without cleansing and purification practices can be debilitating. This might be why you avoid stepping full-time into your healing work or avoid the deeper, more energetic, or shamanic work you are called to do. Having one foot in and one foot out of your sacred work is highly uncomfortable. Cleansing and purification give you access to your more profound work because of the transformation you go through by doing your practices. You might not look or feel like you did before. Get used to letting go, clearing out, and welcoming in intentionally. It will make your life and job a lot easier.

Remember, techniques are amazing; tools are helpful, but your intention and will are the cornerstones, the roots of all you do in this work. Never focus on fear or not being enough. Come from an empowered place. Even though I am telling you how to clean things up, there is no need to be afraid or think twice about what is being cleaned. This is why you spend time building your radiant field and internal reserves. Know you are more than enough and more than capable. Know you are creating an outcome based on what is the highest, best potential—not what you are afraid might happen.

Compassionate Detachment

In particular, you can unknowingly invite in energy by being too attached to the outcome of others' experiences. One way to avoid this is to maintain a sense of compassionate detachment. This means your heart is full of compassion. You show up fully but never pity or aim for a specific outcome because this hooks a cord into the other person's energy body. As a healer and helper, being detached may go against what you've thought. However, your health as a healer depends on the strength of your system, and being overly invested can open you to take on other people's energy, emotions, and even karma as you seek to transmute it.

Be truly present with the other person and what they are experiencing. Ask more questions than make decisions. Inspire possibilities. Awaken this person to their own healer within by being curious and allowing the experience to unfold. Feel into what might be, but allow that you don't know what is to come. In moments of certainty and force, we become rigid, stop listening, and miss the subtle cues that bring more information. In these moments, we need a quick clearing for ourselves because we have moved out of center and placed ourselves too far into the other person.

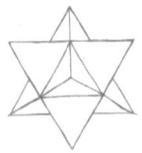

THE LIGHTHOUSE

On the shores of a raging sea, waves crash with
such force that the Earth crumbles.

Seaspray shoots meters up into the air.

The roar is deafening.

The sky is grey and ominous.

On the shore stands a lighthouse.

It is consistent, sturdy, and unmoving.

It takes the waves and gives light,

So that the lost and weary can find their way home.

When you are a master of cleansing and purification, you are a lighthouse.

You stand ready for what you must do; bring light and welcome people home.

Replace that lighthouse with a giant sponge.

The sponge soaks up everything. It has nothing to give back except more of the same of what it has been given, and it sloppily falls into the sea to be washed away.

Be a lighthouse, not a sponge.

2

EMPTYING AND REFILLING

Life is but a constant inhale and exhale.

Cleansing and purification may seem the same, but they are separate processes.

Cleansing includes:

- Moving out what needs to be cleaned up, taken away, let go of.

- The act of purging and releasing.

- Reducing energy in an area.

Purification includes:

- Drawing in new energy, light, love, and beliefs.

- The act of toning or making something stronger, brighter, and more robust.

- Increasing energy in an area.

Cleansing and purification go together because you can't release or remove without drawing in something new. Nature abhors a vacuum. If you remove an energy, block, habit, or thought pattern but don't actively replace it with something new and powerful, you leave an open space for something to enter. It might even be the very thing you spent a lot of time working out of the body and field. After clearing work, bring light and love into the body and field. In belief release work, you clear the belief and replace it with something beneficial. It is easier to change a habit when incorporating a new practice. This gives you somewhere to focus when old desires and patterns come up. We call on light, love, and higher vibrational frequencies to help us.

We are emptying and refilling. This aligns with universal law; there is an exhale and an inhale. If that is not the situation, then you have ceased to exist. Always see how to refill what is empty. If you only fill and add without removing toxic energy, you can do a disservice—giving energy and life force to something that needs clearing.

This is especially important when working with tumors and cancer. You don't want to give the disease more energy; you want to clear and starve it while supporting the rest of the system so the body's natural healing abilities do their job. If you overstimulate energy to the heart, when someone has hypertension or anxiety, you can increase the energy that needs to be brought down and smoothed out. These are subtle awarenesses built upon the intake with your client and your ability to feel and sense energy in their body.

Knowing numerous cleansing and purification practices is vital because you'll have more tools to offer. The best thing you can do as a healer is empower your clients to heal themselves, giving them tools to work with at home. If they do small, regular things, they will advance more quickly and be in a better place for your next session, making your job that much easier.

It fascinates me that so many modalities create a vast power imbalance where the practitioner does things to the person, the person goes away, lives their life, and then has to keep coming back. It sets up a system where the practitioner is now the savior, and the client is the victim, which is disempowering. In one healing school I attended, a business section focused on how to get people coming back week after week, forever. This, the presenter said, was how to be successful. No, thank you! I have always gotten less joy from working with people with this "fix me!" mentality. I believe in empowering my people to do their work, advance quickly, and move on from my care. I want them to have a full toolbox, so they know they can handle life's challenges. Plus, when enabled, they love bringing back reports that they did something that worked!

Willingness to Create Change

As a healer, you must begin with yourself and release energetic baggage, old stories, possessions, and anything else standing in your way. If you are willing to release, then you can make a change.

Many people want their lives to be different: to make more money, have more energy, find a partner, etc. Yet, new actions and ways of being need space to enter. They have no place to come in because their lives, energy bodies, and homes are full of the past. To let go and release can be frightening. We are confronted with our fear of lack. We are afraid that if we release who we are, we may not like what we find on the other side. This requires learning to trust in surrender, the only spiritual practice. You must surrender to the possibility that what you bring in will support you more than what you hold onto now.

Healing is about actively seeking change, and here are some powerful words to initiate this change:

"I am willing. I am willing to let go of what does not serve my highest and best from my body. I am willing to let go of what does not serve my highest and best from my auric field. I am willing to let go of that which does not serve my highest and best from my life."

"I release that which does not serve my highest and best from my body. I release that which does not serve my highest and best from my auric field. I release that which does not serve my highest and best from my life."

You can get really specific about what you are willing to change:

> "I am willing to let go of thoughts, habits, and actions that hold me back from my soul's purpose."

> "I am willing to let go of relationships that keep me stuck in dysfunctional patterns and beliefs."

> "I am willing to let go of constructed identities that no longer serve my evolution and growth."

These phrases are keys to doors locked for years or even lifetimes. Used regularly in your personal practice, you will find that issues you have been "working on" resolve and come up for review in new ways. Notice what arises in you as you read these statements. Do all the sentences feel the same, or are you more worried about one of them working? Could this be a clue that you have been avoiding change?

While cleaning up your body and field, you must look at other areas of your life. How is your home? Your treatment room? Your car? Are there stacks of old papers and bills, dust bunnies, and cobwebs in the corners? When did you last clean the closets or under the bed? Are you holding onto energy from past relationships by keeping things as constant reminders and energetic reservoirs? Do you have a cord to an old life by refusing to give up those office work clothes in case this healer thing doesn't work out? Are your crystals dusty, your altar flowers dead, or is something lurking in the back of the fridge? Are your files and finances in order? Are there aspects of your relationships that need to be cleaned up?

JOURNAL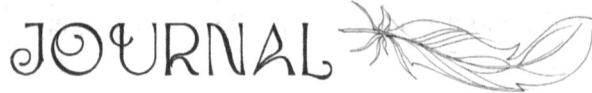

Think about the above list, and journal your answers to the following questions:

- How can I live in greater alignment with what I am calling in?

- How do I feel energetically and emotionally in my living and workspace?

- What needs to be cleaned up?

- What conversation or subtle shift could help raise the place's or situation's vibrational frequency if it can't be changed?

The Empath Misconception

Many support groups and materials exist to help people survive the world as empaths. They generally agree that empaths can feel others' emotions strongly. Most of the time, issues arise because they also take on others' emotions and experience them in their body as their own or as overwhelming and distracting energy. This is different from empathy, a way of "standing in someone else's shoes," seeing and feeling from another's perspective, and having compassion for people even if we can't fully understand what they are going through. Everyone can practice empathy. Not everyone is an empath. Not all empaths can engage fully with empathy, as feelings overwhelm them, and they can't put themselves in someone else's place.

This is because emotions have energy. They leave the body and go out into the world. They pick up energies of the same resonance and then return. There are collective fields of emotions that are contagious. Empaths often suffer from a form of emotional contagion. This can be overwhelming and create illness, shutdown, or inability to cope with the outside world. Many think the only solutions are to shield, block, avoid, and blame.

Some people are natural empaths, but it is also trained during childhood by consistently managing emotions and energies in an unstable or unsafe home. But also, the feelings of the empath are so strong and overwhelming due to resonance with the repressed, constricted emotions stored in the body. When we look at this, it makes sense. If our childhood home is unsafe, we learn how to feel and suck up emotions from others. At the same time, personal emotions aren't fully expressed, seen, and moved through. If we haven't fully felt, accepted, and expressed our pain, it is highly triggering when we come in contact with this in others. We are overwhelmed not only by the emotional field of the other person but also by the resonating energy stuck in our organs and energy field. This trigger could be seen as an experience of a heightened sensation trying to help us tap into and release our repressed emotions. But, instead of looking at it this way, most declare themselves a victim to others' horrible energies and retract from or react to the world.

When you are in right relationship with your feelings and have dealt with repressed emotions from childhood, you can experience others' emotions, but they are more like signals and waves moving through. They give information and then move on. Nothing in your field or body resonates with the energy moving through the environment. Intensity is felt when outside emotional energy confronts stagnant internal energy, creating a larger field of emotion. When you are clearer overall, you can still feel these emotions in others and use them to help you navigate the world or receive information in healing work. But they aren't triggering, exhausting, and debilitating.

You aren't just trying to protect yourself. You are committed to moving repressed and stagnant energies so you aren't as resonant with toxicity from other people and can be a clear vessel for your work. Through this process of cleansing and purification, you raise your vibration, energetic capacity, and ability to move energy more proficiently as needed.

Spiritual OCD

Without meaning to contradict, let me throw out a warning. Stop working on yourself so much. Obsessive-Compulsive Disorder (OCD) is marked by an obsessive need to do things such as counting, hand washing, or locking a door. Sometimes, we go overboard when we begin to understand energy and potential contamination. This can cause us to become fearful, worried, and overly cautious. If you feel overwhelmed, take deep breaths in through the nose with long, slow exhales out of the mouth (to reactivate the parasympathetic nervous system). Remind yourself that you are safe. You are learning essential tools, but your inner stability and trust give them power. This is why we activated and energized the central channel and built the field in the first two chapters, so you have trust in yourself and your internal power. This isn't about adding busy work and spiritual hoops to jump through, which, if not done correctly, will place you in mortal danger.

JOURNAL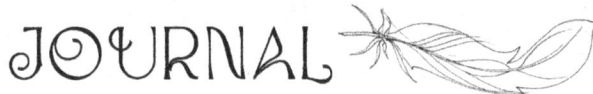

Do any of these statements resonate with you?

- I fear opening my channel, getting close to others in pain, or working with others because I might "pick something up."

- I have felt psychic attacks in the past and shut down the ability to see, hear, or feel to protect myself.

- I fear that if I work on someone, energy might get stuck in my system, and I won't know what to do.

- I forget to cleanse myself, my tools, and my space before or after sessions.

- I am called to pull things out of people's bodies or fields, but I am unsure what to do after that or if this is safe.

- I don't trust my ability to be clear, safe, or protected.

- I have to do cleansing practices all the time, or I am in danger (Spiritual OCD).

- I am afraid I am not powerful enough to deal with certain energies.

3

TOOLS FOR CLEANSING

Clarity arises as much from energetic
clearing as from mental discovery.

Here are cleansing tools you can utilize in your personal practice and before and after client sessions:

Movements: Pulling, moving, tapping, sweeping, grabbing, dragging, and flicking move energy out, off, and away.

Swipes: Before, during, and after sessions, grab and pull energy from your head, face, neck, and body in swiping motions. At the end of the movement, flick the energy off of your hand into the Earth, an imagined fire, a running body of water, or light from above. These portals move energy away from you and your client and into transmutation areas. In the following chapters, we will go over working with the elements and portal creation; these practices will become more precise and personal to you. This creates a new level of presence. You start fresh, free from your thoughts and what you have seen, heard, taken in, and said. The throat and back of the neck are essential. Also, sweep and pull off the arms, kidney area, and down the legs. Quickly flicking your wrist and hand will help get energy off during a session.

Tapping: Use your palms, fingertips, or soft fists to tap and move energy. Tap down your arms and hands, and then feel the energy draining out your fingertips. Use this all over the body; I do extensive tapping practices on my whole body daily. If energy is stuck in a particular area, such as the heart or other organ, tap and pull it out the nearest extremity.

Spiral: The spiral opens an area so energy can be moved out with your hands and breath. Move whatever part of your body you are working to the left in a counter-clockwise motion to open. When you are finished cleansing, go the opposite direction to draw in for purification. This is especially helpful in releasing stuck energy from the hips, diaphragm, and heart during your personal practice. Use the spiral with your hands and fingers during session work to open an area and get energy moving. Then, use pulling, grabbing, dragging, and sweeping to keep the energy moving out. End with a flick to discharge the energy from your hand.

Water: Wash your hands past your elbows after every session in warm water—avoid hot water, which sends energy back up your channels, or cold water unless you're done for the day, as it shuts down energy flowing through your hands. Try using salt with essential oils for extra cleansing.

Sound: I've touched on the importance of using your voice earlier, and this is especially true when releasing and letting go. Sound creates vibrational waves that penetrate your tissues and fields to open and disperse stagnant energy. Emotions are easily released through sound, as when we grieve authentically. Being polite and hiding emotions forces them deep into the body instead of letting them out. Expressing emotions is a challenge for many people who feel ashamed of how it might look or sound. Even in the privacy of our own homes, we may not be comfortable expressing ourselves loudly. However, this is a simple way to release pent-up energy before it becomes stuck in our bodies.

In Medical Qi Gong, we work with sounds for each organ system. These sounds clear stagnant energy and repressed emotions. Below is a chart briefly explaining these organ systems, the sounds used to clear each, and the associated emotions. You will be instructed back to this chart later. There are, of course, other sounds taught by different lineages, systems, and teachers. I'm providing you with sounds to explore, but experiment and use your own natural sounds. When you release them, go with the flow and let your body move intuitively along with the sound.

The organ systems are grouped into sets with a Yin organ and a Yang organ, except for the heart system, a collection of three. Acquired emotions are the ones obtained in this lifetime. They aren't our original essence. We uncover our true, unique selves by clearing out the acquired emotions.

Use this chart to work with cleansing and purifying your body and clients. The critical part of the work is to focus on the vibration in the body. This isn't just sound coming from the vocal cords and throat. The sound vibrates the organs and all through the body. Practice over time will open up the system so that you can feel the vibration moving through you more and more. Let the sounds find the most profound resonance. Explore and elongate the vowels and let the consonants ring. Feel the sound in the body as it gets quieter and into silence. Sound penetrates even when no noise is expressed outwardly.

Element	Yin Organ	Yang Organ	Acquired Emotions	Original Essence	Sound	Color
Metal	Lungs	Large Intestine	Grief Sadness Shame	Confidence Honor Integrity	sss ssh shang	white
Water	Kidneys	Urinary Bladder	Fear Depression Lack of Drive	Determination Focus Wisdom	yu	dark blue dark purple black
Wood	Liver	Gall Bladder	Anger Rage Indecisveness	Compassion Creativity Boundaries	guo	green blue/green
Fire	Heart	Small Intestine Pericardium	Mania Anxiety	Inner Peace Joy	ha	red pink
Earth	Spleen	Stomach	Worry Doubt Rumnination	Trust Surrender Honesty	hung	yellow gold

Breath: The exhale breath releases toxic energy and stuck emotions. You might naturally release forceful breaths from your mouth when you work on yourself or others or in a stressful situation. The body clears itself in many ways, varying from person to person. This includes belching, yawning, sighing, laughing, or crying. Intentionally focusing on the exhale breath helps your system clear more quickly.

Shaking (Frequency Vibration): One of the most profound cleansing practices is shaking, and if you take nothing from this entire book except a shaking practice, you will receive great benefits.

Shaking is an ancient practice, and many cultures found shaking opened them up to spirit. When we open to spirit, which is what awakening is all about, we allow movement of energy, information, and light—which is transformational. Energy has difficulty moving through blockages and holdings in the body. The light doesn't have clear pathways, making it uncomfortable as it pushes through a clogged system. It is the same as a drainpipe. Over the years, a drain will become clogged with residue, bacteria, and the gross stuff you want to pretend doesn't exist. If you never take time to clear the drain and get the nasty stuff broken up and moving, you will end up with a stinky mess.

Shaking clears minor and even large blockages. This practice will support your nervous system as it helps old, unresolved trauma leave the body without having to go into the story that created the contractive force in the physiology. It is the drain cleaner that breaks up stagnation and gets it moving, and it is as simple as shaking every part of the body for a few minutes a day.

[Practice 23: Shaking]

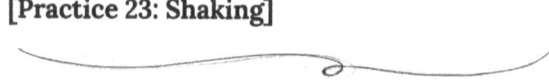

Bring Your Practices Together

As you play with different ways of cleansing, you will feel which you are drawn to, which ones help most, and which are your go-to tools. All of these come together to create a powerful cleansing experience. For example, I might do some shaking with strong exhale breaths out the mouth, then tap my body to find places of tension, pull congested energy out of the arms and other areas, and fling it into the Earth. I will then tap and use my hands and the vibration of tones to address my organs and emotions. I will allow intuitive movement, rocking or spiraling along with sounds, and an emotional release may come up with crying, laughing, or even singing. I then draw my arms up and pull fresh light into my body as I anchor new energy, thoughts, and emotions through purification, as discussed below.

4

PURIFICATION PRACTICES

If you knew how much light you hold, you would be blinded.

After cleansing comes purification—filling in the now open space to raise your vibration and frequency. Reflect on what you can add to your life to make it of a higher vibration and more aligned with who you want to be. Would you like to meditate, pray, drum, sing, or dance more? Are you getting enough vitamins and minerals? Do you crave time with a spiritual teacher or friend? Would building an altar help focus your energy? Ask what you want more of and follow the inspirations that arise. The energy, thoughts, words, and actions you cultivate align with your essence expressed. When these come together, you create significant positive change in your life. Contemplation, followed by action, means you are creating with intention. That is powerful.

Purification is letting in the light; it is an active choice. Do you replenish yourself? Rest, sunshine, good food, and laughter bring in positive energy. Some of us work in dark places and must be nurtured with fun and lightness. Being spiritual and raising your vibration doesn't mean you must always be serious. Being light-filled allows you to be silly, impulsive, and free to dance about in your underpants.

What is your relationship with receiving? Can you luxuriate in it? Can you receive love, touch, care, concern, and appreciation from others without feeling you must give back? Do you feel worthy of the light?

Here is a phrase to help you align with receiving:

"I receive from the Universe, myself, and others with ease. I take nourishment into all my systems without shame, fear, or regret. I allow myself to receive without needing to give in return right away. I allow light to enter my form, bringing me toward greater alignment."

Purification Tools

The following purification tools are all nourishing practices.

Movement: Projecting, infusing, drawing, and pulling in are movements used in purification.

[Practice 24: Projecting Energy]

Sound: Sounds break up and disperse energy in cleansing but can also draw in and soothe. Think of this as bringing harmony. What tones or songs feel harmonizing and nurturing to you? Experiment in your practice and your healing space. The songs or tones you use toward the end of a session should be especially soothing. I tone and sing in my client sessions, and there is a difference in the sounds my client and I make to break up and move energy (cleansing sounds) than when harmonizing toward the end of the session (purification).

Color: Colors tonify (build and fortify) the energy centers, fields, and organs. They draw focused light in. I refer you back to the chart to see the colors that go with the organs. Some people find it easy to connect with, see, or experience colors, while others need their imagination until their inner sight expands. It is beneficial to gently focus on the back base of your skull, specifically the occipital ridge, to enhance your ability to see colors. This means looking as if you can see through the back of your skull while your eyes are soft and relaxed. It does not mean rolling your physical eyes toward the back of your head. Try this while invoking the colors during meditation. Meditate on each color, and spend time with it. Feel it in your body. See how it wants to be used. I am providing some information, but your intuition and knowledge will guide you in choosing the appropriate colors for any situation. You may also be able to read people by colors. You might notice if they seem bright and colorful or dull, dark, or have black areas. This is important in assessing your client's fields, emotions, and health. Again, some find working with colors easy and natural. Others are less connected. I encourage you to try more challenging things and practice what is easy for you.

Breath: The inhaled breath draws in energy. Focus on long, slow inhales as you imagine light or color drawing into your body. Draw in on the inhale and then let it disperse to where it is needed in the body on the exhale. Or draw light in on the inhale and radiate that light out in all directions on the exhale. Again, this purification practice fills, nurtures, and blesses you with light.

[Practice 25: Purifying Breath]

Other Tools for Purifying and Cleansing

Elements: You will connect to the elements more in Chapter 4, The Sacred Container. They can be called upon in session work, such as to burn away or warm (fire), wash away or cool (water), bring in sweet new possibilities and messages (air or wood), or fill you with nurturing Earth energy.

Energetic beings (spirit guides and forces): You will develop better relationships with these in the following two chapters. As you learn about your guides and teachers, call upon them to help move out energy or welcome in something new. This will become clear as we move on.

Prayer and ceremony: Extended presence, devotion, and repetition bring power to your requests and allow your intentions to come into form.

Visualization and affirmation: These connect you to your future self and the most beneficial future outcome for all, creating change in the present moment.

Tools and allies from the natural world: These are the nature spirits of places, trees, crystals, and your other Earth-based connections. You will learn how they support you by building your relationships, asking questions, and experimenting with how they want to collaborate with you. The following two chapters will clarify this.

Cleanse and Purify Energy Systems Instead of Reliving the Story

By using energetic cleansing and purification exercises, you can heal without going into the story behind the energy. This saves time and is less re-traumatizing. You often don't need to go into the story (especially if you have told the story over and over again). We easily attach to stories because the brain is obsessed with creating, knowing, and living in stories. The problem is that the story can keep you living in the past and building a future you don't desire. The stories you tell yourself—from the past or worry about the future, are truths as your brain processes them. Less focus on the story and more on the movement of energy and emotions can allow you to shift ways of being that have been stuck and deal with intense and overwhelming events. This doesn't mean that memories won't surface or that certain things will not need to be voiced and discussed with a professional or friend.

We tend to hook onto stories, memories, emotions, thoughts, and beliefs and hold them close. We like to create identities and structures to live in and repeat the same stories, but this isn't what freedom is all about. Feelings, thoughts, and stories will emerge when you do these practices. It is helpful to see them as passing clouds moving up and through the layers of your body and field. They are leaving, so don't hold onto them through further identification.

[Practice 26: Cleansing and Purification]

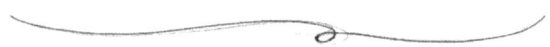

Cleansing and Purifying Clients in Sessions

All the cleansing and purification tools described in this section can be used in client sessions. You learn these tools by working on yourself. Your personal practice teaches you how to use these tools effectively in client sessions.

> **Movement:** Pulling, moving, tapping, sweeping, and flicking can be used in and on the body and through the fields. Shaking, kneading, and pressing can be used in the tissues and energy points to open and move energy. Use the spiral in the counterclockwise direction in the field or even the tissue to open an area and then pull or press energy out. Use the clockwise motion to purify an area, drawing energy in.

> **Breath:** Sync your breath with your client at the beginning of the session, then use your breath to guide them. When working, it is helpful to turn your head to the side and expel

all your breath out of your mouth occasionally. This helps you move the energy and not take it in. You can guide your client through inhaling, gathering breath, and then releasing out the mouth while you move the energy. You may have them hold their breath to collect stagnant energy and then guide them to release it as you work. They may need support finding their breath in their belly as many are chronic chest breathers. This simple instruction and awareness can bring significant benefits.

Sound: You can use sound to break up stagnations and bring harmony while working. You may not be practiced in using sound in sessions, but when you are comfortable making sounds, it gives your client permission to release in this way. If you're working on old stuck energy or a stagnant area, having the client tone and make sound with you is helpful. Even in talk sessions, if they are coming up against something painful, it can help to guide them to make a sound and continue with it until the energy is fully released. They have been denied expression through their voice, so they need permission and guidance. Review the chart to see if any specific sounds support you. Again, simple sighing and the "ha" sound are potent and sometimes all you need. Try to find the sound of an emotion, feeling, or memory. You can support your sound work with bells, rattles, chimes, tuning forks, singing bowls, or other small hand-held instruments. Work with them in your personal practice; they will teach you how to use them in session.

Color: Use colors to purify or enhance after cleansing or releasing an area, organ, or energy center or after an emotional release. Ask your clients to imagine the color with you.

Working with Nature and Utilizing Visualization: In my sessions, I release and remove a lot of negative energies and blockages. I develop relationships with trees and the Earth to help me hold and compost these energies. I also imagine a stream of water under the table moving quickly out into the ocean. I bring my clients into this process by describing this stream so they, too, can imagine any negativity, shadow, tar, or darkness flowing downward into this stream and out into the ocean. I want my clients to become self-sufficient in all things. I want them to be masters of their own healing so they can do this work on themselves when they can't see me. I am a portal, a channel, and a bridge. I am here to help people own their healing and transformation. The more I bring them into the process, the better for me. All people are powerful. All people have access to their own healing system. Why wouldn't I want them to help out and learn how to do this work themselves? This also gives them a focus and removes the fear of releasing toxic energy because they are concerned the practitioner will take it on from them.

[Practice 27: **Releasing Into the Stream**]

[Practice 28: **Final Purification**]

[Practice 29: **Final Purification with a Client**]

5

CARING FOR YOUR HEALING SPACE

You ask Divine Beings to come into your space, and
you haven't bothered to clear the cobwebs?

The treatment room is a sacred place and a direct reflection of your internal spiritual self, so rooting out clutter and areas where energy is discordant is essential. It is helpful if the room has sunlight and fresh air. This isn't always possible, so I encourage you to do what you can with what you have and choose your treatment spaces wisely.

After a treatment, there is energetic residue. You, your client, and your next client will be submerged in it if you don't take care of the space. Emotions, thought forms, trauma, and toxic energy have been released. Watch out for the corners where it likes to collect. If, over a long period, this energy is allowed to accumulate, a negative energetic portal can be created. Beings are looking for food, and you set out a buffet!

Monthly or even weekly deep cleanings are needed. This will depend on the intensity of your work and the space you are treating from. If there is an open door or window into nature, you will have an easier time than if you are stuck in a closed room in an office building. You should also do more clearings if you have the healing space in your home. I used to treat from my living room and was vigilant about clearing before and after every client. Clearing before was important because I didn't want to affect the session's energy with my personal life.

Every time you do healing work, you open the container for Divine beings to come and assist you. Opening to the other realms holds the possibility that other beings will also show up. This is why closing the container, which we will discuss more in the next chapter, and regular cleaning up is essential.

Cleansing Tools

There are many ways to cleanse your space, but your intention is your most essential tool.

> **Creating a portal:** Remember that energy needs a place to go. It is helpful to get into the practice of opening and closing a cleansing portal for your work. The basics of creating a portal are that after preparing yourself energetically for your session, use your hand and intention to open a portal for energy to leave the space. Use the counterclockwise motion to open the portal to a helpful ally for you. This could be to the divine light above, the center of the Earth below, or into fire or water. Be sure to close the portal (clockwise motion) at the end of the session.

[Practice 30: Creating a Portal]

> **Tools and allies:** You can use a spray or smudge. You can buy purifying sprays of sage, lavender, or other herbs. You can also create one using purified water, alcohol (vodka), essential oils, and adding in other magical ingredients as you feel called, such as gem elixirs, flower essences, tiny crystals, and even salt. Set your intentions into the spray as you make it, and offer prayers and gratitude. Many herbs and woods are burned for cleansing and bringing in new energies. You may have been introduced to sage, palo santo, and sweetgrass. While these are common tools of Western practitioners, please be aware that over-harvesting is a real problem with these sacred herbs. Only buy from places that consider their environmental impact. I

prefer to grow my own herbs for smudge sticks or burning on charcoal or to work with my local wild plants such as juniper or cedar. This means I work with more local herbs and have complete control over how they are grown and the intentions put into their production, and I am not depleting precious resources. I get to know the herbs personally, make offerings when I plant and harvest them, and discover how they want to work, as they will be more attuned to cleansing, purification, or specific healings or rituals. I also get to work with plants that are more sacred to my lineage instead of borrowing from the traditions of others. Experiment. Sit with these powerful allies and feel what is right for your work.

Cleansing and purification movements: As I described in the previous section, you can use pulling, moving, sweeping, and flicking motions with your hands to clear a room. Clap your hands to clear the space. This also wakes the healing centers in your hands where the energy flows. Hold hands up, palms out, allow yourself to push, and rake the air. As you move along, feel the places where the energy feels stagnant. It might feel like thickness that requires you to slow down or go over the area again. Imagine light emanating from your hands as you do this. Push the energy around in a circle through the room and out a door or window. Experiment with what works for you, and always ask for help from your guides. Use your hands to soothe and brighten the room at the end, pulling in and down beneficial energy.

Light and color: Many people find calling in and using the violet ray, imagining it burning away any discordant energies, helpful. You can use other colors as you are intuitively called. Fill yourself with light and then radiate it into the room, filling the space with light to complete the purification after cleansing what is no longer needed.

Sound: Clapping, whistles, and sharp and loud sounds break up energy and get it moving. You can direct energy to move with chimes, drums, bowls, or bells. A cooking pot and wooden spoon work well in a pinch. This creates an energetic distortion that breaks up energy, disrupting the forms of spirit entities that prefer to be in the dark and quiet. Complete by playing beautiful music to re-harmonize. Fill the space with your song.

Trees: Whenever possible, work with a healer tree you have connected with beforehand. Ask the tree if it will help the healing process, and tell it what you would like its assistance doing. If it is open to the task, you can work with this tree to help pull the energy down into the Earth. You should also determine the closest large body of water to direct energy into the water as you clear. If you don't have a tree nearby, I recommend creating a relationship with a large old tree near you. Visit it often, make offerings at its base, and talk to it. These might be cornmeal (or your local or lineage grain), tobacco, or special herbs. You might leave bird seed and water for the animals this tree supports. Sit in meditation with this tree. Ask for its assistance on your healer's path. You can call on this tree in session if you are cycling a lot of energy that feels like it should go down into the earth. If this is not possible, imagine your favorite type of tree, connect with its essence, and work with the spirit of the tree. You will learn more about developing these relationships in the next chapter.

Potted Plants: Plants are excellent allies as they suck up toxic energy in the healing room as they cycle and clean the air. They will thrive in a healing space. Plants generally ground toxic energy through their roots into the earth. If they are in pots, it can be helpful to take them outside occasionally so they can have contact with the earth (even if it is through the pot). If taking them outside is impossible, I recommend watering your plants with blessed water or placing a stone or crystal in the pot. Ask the crystal to collect any harmful energy and then cleanse that crystal outside or in other ways that I will discuss in the cleansing and charging crystals section.

Prayer and ceremony: Use prayer to help with your cleansing process. Prayer connects you to your heart and higher guides and often inspires the perfect words and intentions to emerge. When you enter a new space or leave one, a ceremony to honor all the spirits of the land, spirits of the space (or home), and the Earth, and to call in your guides to the new healing space is helpful. When entering a new space, you want to cleanse and purify it before doing work there.

Visualization and affirmation: Once again, your imagination is integral to your experience. If you feel guided intuitively, follow that. Visualize the space clearing. Let your mind's eye find darkness and move it, sending it through your portal. Affirm for yourself: This space is now clean and clear.

Elements: Throw energy into a candle flame or a fire of your imagination. Water also cleanses and moves things out. Air blows through, breaking up stagnant energies and bringing in fresh breath. Earth is an excellent composter, and you can send energy into it. We will discuss the elements more in The Sacred Container.

Burning salt: Another great cleansing technique I like a lot is putting salt on a heat-safe dish and adding rubbing alcohol. I use a cast iron cauldron for this with a heat-resistant cork pad underneath. You can also use a thick ceramic dish. It will get hot, so make sure it is heat-safe. Pinch the salt into a pile if it falls and set it on fire using a long-handled lighter or long match for safety, letting it burn in the room until it goes out. This will produce smoke, so be aware if you have smoke detectors nearby. Also, this is fire and an accelerant. Please be aware that it might make a larger flame than you intended. Start small and use caution. Do not leave it unattended. Do not get the alcohol on your body, clothes, or the surrounding area; make sure you are not near flammable materials. Have ventilation but not a windy area. Be cautious of pets, and don't show this to children, as they might take it upon themselves to experiment without realizing the dangers. Dispose of the salt, flushing it down the toilet. This technique strongly pulls negative energy into the salt and transmutes it.

After cleansing, use purification techniques to balance the area and fill it with light. Incorporate all the same systems: color, light, harmonizing sounds, and your powerful intention to bring in and fill the space with light, love, and healing. Project energy and light to fill the space, use colors to achieve your desired effect, play harmonious music, and burn sweet and fragrant resins and herbs. Place fresh flowers in the room.

Crystal Cleansing and Charging

Crystals are powerful allies. However, to utilize their full potential, they must be cleansed and purified. You can call upon other allies to support you in this endeavor. For instance, I rely on the soothing flow of creeks to cleanse my crystals. Consider which of your allies can help you with this process.

Stones with lunar energy, such as moonstone or selenite, prefer cleansing and charging under the full moon. Stones with sun quality, like citrine or amber, prefer the sun. Magical tools rely on the alignment of relationships and correspondences, so providing them with similar energy for support will enhance your work with them. Another method is to place them in salt water overnight or for up to a week for a complete clearing and then onto the Earth for three days, where green grows.

Just as you follow cleansing with purification, it's important to finish clearing with programming. Ground yourself by standing or sitting and connecting to the Earth. Draw energy up into your belly and hold the crystal in your left hand. With your right hand, energetically activate it with a clear and precise function. Feel the energy of your intention moving through your body and out of your hand. Hold it up to the Divine and ask for additional support and blessings. You can sing to the crystal, meditate with it, and focus on its purpose.

They say a dog isn't happy without a job. The same is true for crystals. I actively engage with them by listening deeply and assigning them specific tasks to fulfill for a period of time. Some crystals are programmed for particular clients and intended to help with specific issues or to enhance certain aspects of their being. Others help me read people, perform psychic surgery, clear energy from a room, or awaken a specific chakra. If you listen, you will discover their preferred area of expertise. In a crystal shop, I ask to be led to the one that wants to do a specific function, such as clearing, extracting, soothing, grounding, etc. Sometimes, I can sense a stone's intended purpose upon picking it up. However, there are instances when I only discover its purpose after working with it for some time.

It's important to note that certain crystals, like Selenite, should not be submerged in water. Similarly, some, like Amethyst, may fade in sunlight, so it's best to research before exposing them to these elements. Kyanite and black tourmaline are self-cleaning and do not require any special techniques. Shungite, one of my favorite healing stones, is black but recharges best in the sun.

Some people keep their 'working crystals' covered when not in use. Again, experiment to see what feels right to you. I also like to awaken the crystals' energies by saying: "Wake up crystal and stone beings. Thank you for your service. Please let your desire to work in the session be known and obvious."

I use various tools, such as flower essences, essential oils, stones, drums, rattles, feathers, skins, and other items I have collected. At the beginning of my work, I invite them to wake up and play with me as they feel called. I then actively listen during sessions to hear when they ask to be brought forward. This is a practice of surrendering to the flow of the moment and the nudges that come in your work and following these inspired instructions. Explore different healing tools, receive training from experts, and use journey work to connect with the frequency of each item. Once you are confident in their use, incorporate them into your sessions. These tools may include chimes, singing bowls, or any items mentioned earlier. Continuously broadening your understanding and collection of tools keeps your work stimulating and engaging for you and your clients.

While tools and helpers can be useful in your work, don't lose sight of your own true ability. Neither the paraphernalia nor the clothes make the shaman. They are helpful team members but don't get lost in them.

[Practice 31: Collector Crystal in Water]

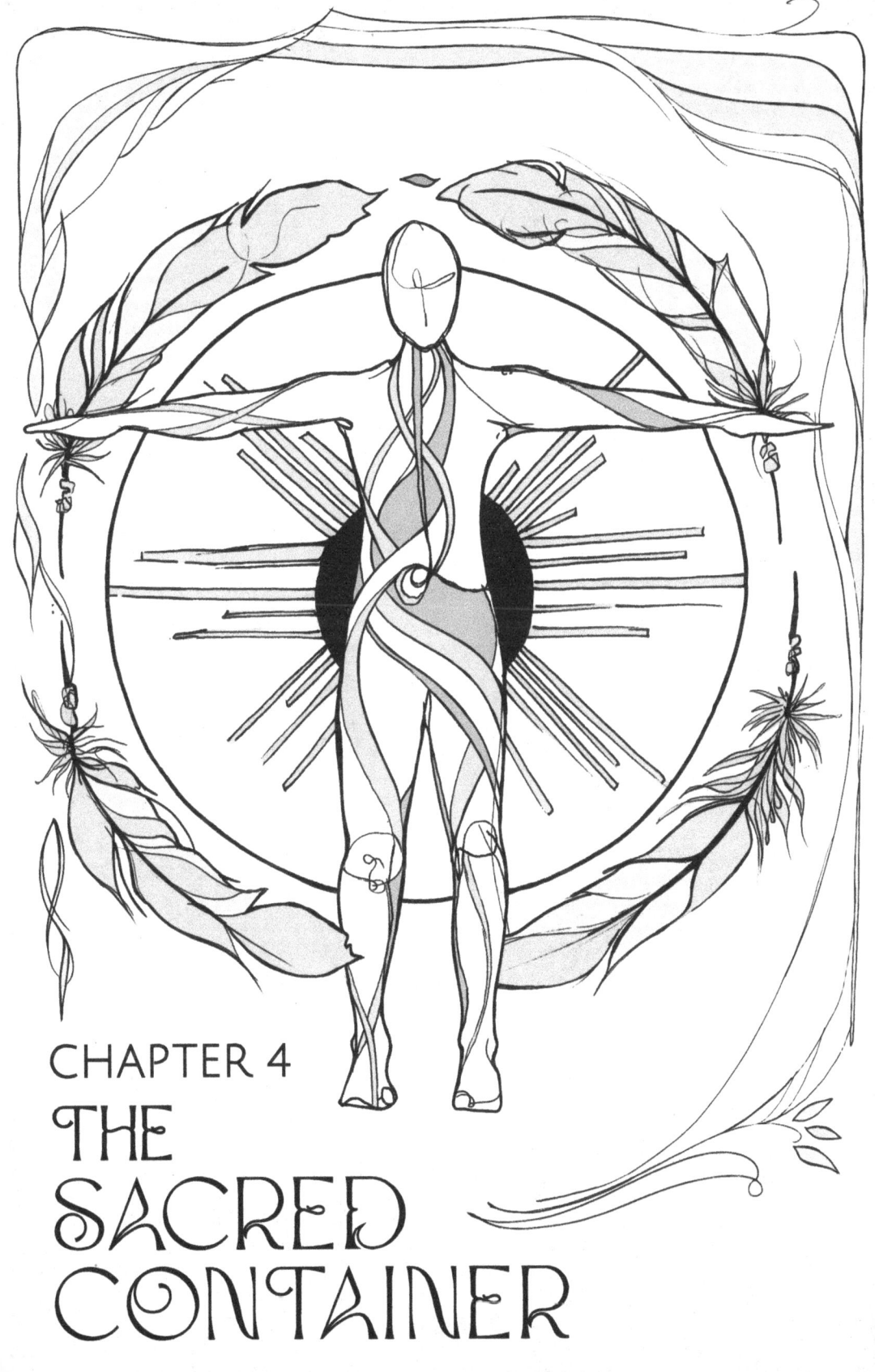

CHAPTER 4
THE
SACRED
CONTAINER

CHAPTER 4

THE SACRED CONTAINER

The sacred container builds on the previous chapters because you want to be in a place of full, radiant power before interacting with other energies. Only once you are solid within yourself and your field and able to feel, track, and move energy should you stretch out to work with others. From this empowered presence, you'll use the tools you learned in the previous chapters to build your sacred container, which resonates with your field and is linked to your core and connection to the above and below. You are now clear, present, and capable enough to begin this larger work.

The topics in this chapter include:

- Identifying the energies supporting you and your work.

- Working with guides, spirits, elements, directions, and animals.

- Opening and closing a safe, sacred space for healing, meditation, or channeling.

- Feeling guided, protected, and assisted.

- Building functional invocations for spiritual support.

1

ENERGETIC BOOKENDS

Healing happens in a carefully crafted container.

We have explored how the healer's process involves building relationships: to your "I AM," your sovereignty, purpose, intrinsic gifts, and awareness. From there, you moved outward and built relationships with energy fields, the Earth, and celestial energies. Then, you explored how to work with external energies, both light and dark, by understanding them and utilizing practices and tools for cleansing and purification. In this chapter, you'll continue to develop your relationships, but this time with guides, spiritual beings, and other energies—including the inner healer, shaman, medicine person, or whatever word you resonate with.

A note on these titles. The term "shaman" comes from the Siberian Tungus word "saman" and has its roots in Northern Siberia. However, it has been widely adopted as a universal term to describe a consistent role found in intact cultures worldwide. It's worth mentioning that different cultures have different titles for this role, and some individuals may also identify themselves with titles others may not recognize. I use the terms "shaman" and "shamanic" because we can now agree on this vital role in a community. They are the ones who know, the ones who move between the worlds, and the ones who aid the community and communicate with the spirit realms. They are initiated and recognized first and foremost by the spirits and then by their community. There are also many forms of shamanic practitioners, depending on the work they do and their level of abilities.

We all have animistic and shamanic roots in our lineages. Animism is the belief that everything has a spiritual essence and is animated and alive. It acknowledges the importance of social relationships with non-human beings, including animals, plants, rocks, and other entities of the environment. Animism and shamanism are words used by anthropologists in an attempt to label what is widely held and inherent to most indigenous peoples. Before religion and persecution, people from every corner of the planet were deeply connected to nature and the spirit worlds, and a calling toward this role would have been supported and nurtured. You have indigenous roots originating from cultures that utilized shamanic tools to enter trance states, speak with spirits, travel in the unseen realms, incorporate spirits, and bring healing. To be our authentic selves, we do not need to copy and take on another's culture; we need to awaken within ourselves what is natural.

It is vital to consider the impacts of our language and tendencies to appropriate from other cultures. This is why many avoid the word shaman for a Western practitioner. After much reflection, I have come to peace with this word and seek to honor its origin point and all those who hold this sacred title, though I generally use the term shamanic to describe myself instead of shaman. While other cultures have their individual terms for these types of individuals, Western people have lost theirs and so borrow this word. It is not ideal to use a word derived from when an anthropologist experienced the unbroken lineage of a specific shamanic individual and community. But, because the study of these types of healers is extensive, we can agree on what one means when we use this particular word. Consider that unless Western people embrace and stand in this role for our people, indigenous healers are forced to lift the load of the Western world and practice outside their communities that deserve their presence. Western people suffer from the broken threads of our ancient ancestors. Still, we can reweave these threads and stand with our indigenous siblings to bring Earth-based wisdom and healing to the world.

I also believe it is important to consider these titles because, as you discovered in the section on archetypes, there are shadow aspects to consider. Shamans work with spiritual power and cultivate relationships with spirits and power allies of the natural world. When one walks this path, the ego and desire for more power or influence can create negative bonds resulting in harm. The amount of force one has to heal can be used to harm. If we are unwilling to look at the seriousness of this path by diminishing our words, we risk falling toward corruption.

Why the Modern Practitioner Needs Additional Support

In many traditions, when working with a healer or shaman, family and community hold a healing space for the person, using heart energy to feed the process. In this collective experience, the shaman isn't creating the energy but orchestrating or focusing it. The shaman speaks between the worlds, brings information, and clarifies the issues. But the energy of the collective helps the soul to draw back into the body, the person to become whole again, and the healing to occur.

In some traditions, shamans work in groups, traveling through realms together, while others drum, rattle, sing, and stoke the fire. Family members are present and pray for their loved ones. In some cultures, the entire village is present for days to support a lost soul returning home. Many shamans and Indigenous healers spend days preparing to see a client and then treating them. The person doesn't go home until the process is complete.

We have become a world of one healer in one room with one client, often working for an hour or maybe two. In this section, I help you understand how to call upon the additional energy and support you need.

Bookends

The sacred container bookends a session. The work you do is the story in between. If the bookends are present, the story is stable and supported. The sacred container provides structure, safety, and protection. It establishes the tone and intention of the work and offers clear, easily defined parameters for spiritual support.

Held in the container, the client feels supported and safe to be with their challenging stories. Their energy body tracks what is occurring even if they aren't consciously aware of it. A solid container helps them relax and surrender to the experience. Their guides, higher self, and specific beings will be invited into the space to do the healing work. Too much chaos isn't conducive to healing. The container brings focus. The more you create the container, the faster and more relaxed your healing work.

When creating or closing the container, enter into reverence and devotion. Use everything you have learned so far: coming home to yourself, sourcing, and heightening your awareness. You have already cleansed and purified yourself and your space. From this place, you are powerful in the construction of the container. It is a tangible experience that you and your client are participating in.

What Energies Are Connected to Your Work?

It's up to you to determine the energies connected to your work. Even if someone suggests you're linked to a specific deity or energy or pulls a card with an animal on it, it's ultimately your responsibility to identify what resonates, what's consistent, and what's genuine.

The work you are called to do already has its own frequency and beings supporting it. It is important to remember that you're not alone in your work. Your spiritual support team wants to be involved and bless you with power, inspiration, and support. Often, they are simply waiting for you to ask for help. Self-work, meditation, and journaling help the connected energies make themselves known. Trust this life-long journey as it unfolds in deepening waves of clarity over time.

As you get to know a guide, you can connect with this energy by devoting an altar to it. You might include colored fabrics, crystals, images, and objects representing your connection. Honor and contribute to the relationship. Talk to them about your work, your mission, and what you need for it to be manifest, successful, and profound. You can even ask for help building your client base. We have already done work around your core why and intention. Use what you have discovered to envision the world you want to live in, feel the energy of it, and then ask for help and guidance.

It's natural to hope for quick and clear answers to all your questions, but connecting with guides is often a subtle experience. They may communicate in colors, sensations, or intuitive insight. They might convey messages through symbols, single words, or mental images. They might even be speaking to you in synchronicities in your life that you are currently ignoring. It may take time to establish a consistent connection. To enhance your process, focus on your intention, make your requests, and then try to remain calm and present, allowing the connection to unfold.

Here are phrases you can use to get started:

- "I commit to the mission of . . . I ask the highest energies that serve this mission to come into my awareness and make themselves known. Thank you for allowing me to do this work."

- "I call upon my healing guide to know you more fully. I ask that you be present with me as I work on . . ."

- "Thank you for easily bringing the people connected to this work, those who need my medicine, into my life."

2

SETTING YOUR COMPASS

May the purest light guide and lead me to my highest path.

This chapter helps you tune into and know your spiritual guides and teachers. While this work is valid and helpful, it is essential to understand who you serve. This means recognizing who you are and your relationship with a higher power. This might be God/Goddess, a specific lineage, or a pure connection to Source, Light, or the Dao.

An adage is, "If you don't stand for something, you'll fall for anything." You have to know what you stand for in your spiritual work. Many seek the spiritual realms but haven't healed their relationship with Source energy or a higher power. Wounds of religion and society often damage this essential bond. When we engage with spirits, we interact with beings who, despite their advanced natures, have yet to attain the highest levels. They may still possess agendas and desires and have limited viewpoints. Focusing solely on these realms and ignoring a higher connection can hinder your progress.

What is your understanding of the ultimate expression of light and love at its highest frequency? This is an inquiry only you can step into. It isn't something anyone else can provide. This is your connection to the ultimate, the limitless. Your inner compass is your guiding principle and awakened sense of higher service. It acts as a safety net, providing direction and holding you accountable. Anything that doesn't align with your inner compass is not on your path.

Higher Self and Oversoul

Developing a bond with your higher self or oversoul is crucial. This aspect of your being is your eternal consciousness, unencumbered by the acquired elements of this lifetime. It grants you access to your spiritual connection to Source energy and all that there is. Connection to the higher self is cultivated through quieting and stilling your logical mind, which may otherwise warp and shift messages received. When you establish a strong relationship with your higher self, the ego's desire for control and input diminishes.

Communication from your higher self can be easy to overlook, as it is subtle. However, it is essential to connect with it intentionally to benefit from its guidance. By learning to sense its presence and practicing listening to your wisdom self, you can develop your ability to receive its messages.

The less-used term "oversoul" refers to an all-encompassing, eternal aspect that oversees everything you do. Connecting with this aspect is crucial because it allows you to receive messages and information more clearly and makes communicating with other spirit beings easier. Your oversoul is a member of a family of beings that exist across different timelines, planets, and dimensions, including the space between lifetimes. By tapping into your oversoul, you can connect with other beings with similar soul signatures. It feels like these entities are akin to your siblings or cousins, making communication with them easier. This also connects you to your soul lineage and may contribute to your attraction to specific places, times, or types of beings. Communicating via your higher self or oversoul gives you access to greater safety and sustainability in these works. It helps you make better decisions in your daily life based on this higher input and intuitive awareness.

To strengthen your spiritual connection, believe in yourself and have faith. Doubt, fear, disbelief, and hopelessness weaken this connection. Fear and doubt are the primary obstacles to spiritual growth. It is normal to doubt spiritual experiences, but don't let fear or skepticism hold you back from pursuing development.

Understand that doubt often arises from societal conditioning and an inner feeling of unworthiness. You are a spiritual being capable of spiritual experiences simply because you exist.

It is essential to have pure intentions when seeking a connection to the spiritual realms. If your motivation is to feed your ego or take advantage of others, you will hinder this connection. While you may connect with other beings, you will not be congruent with your higher self, which can lead to delusions of grandeur and pathological behavior. Confront yourself to see if you have a hidden agenda. Do you want to be special more than you want to be of service? You must also avoid trying to manipulate or alter the messages you receive. Instead, surrender yourself to a higher will, even if it conflicts with what you've learned in the past. This can be difficult for the ego and rational mind, which crave control and personal gain.

[Practice 32: Connecting to Your Higher Self]

3

INVOCATION

*The presence of spiritual support is available
to everyone, but not everyone asks for it.*

Invocation is a call to a guide, teacher, being, energy, or deity to
be with you—a request for presence. You can then inform why the
presence is being asked for, creating greater clarity. It is essential
to be clear about whom you are invoking. For example, if you want
healing for yourself or others and know that Archangel Raphael is
connected to healing, you may call upon him. You may call upon
the Buddha if you seek peace in your heart. If you are working on
compassion and forgiveness, you may want to connect to Mother
Mary or Quan Yin, the Goddess of Compassion and Mercy.

You may also be unsure of whom to call upon. In these cases,
you can send out a more generalized invocation. Here are some
examples of this invocation process.

- "I call upon and invoke the presence of Archangel Raphael to
  assist in this highest of healings."

- "I call upon and invoke the presence of Mother Mary to teach
  me about compassion, forgiveness, and love. I struggle with
  forgiveness and ask to be bathed in your radiant light."

- "I call upon and invoke the presence of my highest of guides
  and teachers to be present with me in my meditation today.
  Allow me to receive illumination from your wisdom."

- "I call upon and invoke the presence of my guardian angel as I am feeling fear and lack of safety. Please guide my steps and illuminate my decisions with your light."

From this, you have created a sacred container in that your space is in the presence of a divine being. This container is for healing, prayer, or meditation. Always be grateful and thank this being for their support. You will learn more about releasing the energies in the section Closing the Container.

You can use the following invocation to call in a larger guiding force.

"Welcome, welcome, welcome. I call, I call, I call upon and invoke the presence of the angels, the archangels, the ascended masters and guides, all those known and unknown that assist and support the work of the light. I call only those that serve my highest and best, only those that serve the light. I welcome you into this space for the purpose of healing and transformation. I ask that you be known to me as needed and that all work be processed with grace and ease. I call upon Source, Divine Light, to be present in this space."

For session work, as you call in the energies, it is helpful to add the name of the person you are working with. "I call upon and invoke Source presence, the guides, angels, and beings of light, doctor and teacher spirits of myself and [insert name] along with our higher selves to assist in this highest of healings for [insert name]."

Or, "I welcome all guides and beings of light that serve [insert name] to come into this space to help this person heal and evolve. Thank you for your assistance."

To show appreciation for the energies you work with, place small bowls on your altar and add offerings. This symbolizes payment for the help and support received and honors the reciprocal nature of your relationship. Acknowledge the presence and energy of the being with gratitude and appreciation. At the end of a healing, spiritual connection, or prayer session, it is polite to thank and release the energies you have called upon. This helps to close the container at the end. You may want to anchor this with a physical movement such as Pulling Down the Heavens or by singing a song. After completion, place the offerings near a tree you work with and say a prayer.

4

THE DIRECTIONS

*I am centered in the directions. They nurture
me with their wisdom and blessings.*

As you work with the directions, you tap into a grid of support, grounding your perception and skills in a geometric field beyond yourself. When we began The Healer's Process, you were guided to build your inner column of light, which reaches into the above and below. You then built the field around your body. Now, you are anchoring that column and energy body into the grids and fields of the earth. She has an energy body much like yours, with a central channel in the form of the main pole through the planet and channels such as the equator, which corresponds with your belt channel, which runs around your belly. Her energy fields contain information in the same way that yours do. Expand your awareness to include these grids or channels of the earth so you can experience these potent currents and work with them for protection, power, and cultivation of specific energies.

Traditions and perspectives worldwide vary regarding the correspondence of directions and entities. You can study different lineages and look up correspondence charts in books or online. Even better, sit facing each direction, build an altar, and observe who and what connects with you from that direction. Explore your local environment on foot and by map to discover what influencing energies inhabit the land around you. Where are the mountains, ocean, or rivers? How does water and, therefore, energy move through the land?

Your spiritual work can be informed by those who have come before, but it is deeply rooted in your own experience. Working with the directions and their corresponding energies shows respect for everything that exists and acknowledges the flow of life of which you are a part. This is your practice and the relationships you are developing. Allow yourself to meditate and play in the directions to find what resonates.

Start with the energetics of the directions as you experience them. Think of the cycles of energies that move through them. In one direction, the sun rises, and in the opposing one, it sets. This also means that another direction contains the sun's energy at its zenith, and the opposing one holds the night's energy. Each direction also corresponds to seasons, elements, animals, plants, minerals, and beings of the unseen realms. Ask yourself, What are the energetic essences that I experience here? Who and what shows up in my awareness when considering this direction?

As you develop these correspondences and build your relationships, your practice honors the directions, elements, and beings of these directions through your invocations and gratitude.

In *The Healer's Process Practice Manual*, I explain two forms of directional invocations and practices for deepening this powerful ritual in your work.

[Practice 33: Calling in the Directions]

5

ANIMAL GUIDES

May I never forget that I, too, am an animal.
And, often, other animals are wiser than I.

Many people have special connections with certain animals, often stemming from an unexplainable feeling of belonging. When I was a child, I was obsessed with animals. I spent hours poring over animal information cards. Eventually, I cut out the animals and covered an entire wall of my room. At nine, I felt such a deep connection with animals that I became a vegetarian. Today, animals are my guides and teachers, providing me with a comforting, supportive presence in my life and work. My animal guides interweave their medicine with mine. Their wisdom and abilities deeply influence my work.

Animal guides are powerful allies and can be significant life-long relationships. Their energy is easily accessible and beneficial. Many would never dare to traverse into the spirit world without the assistance and protection of their animal guide. When you are blessed with this meaningful connection, honor it through conversation, images on your altar or in your home, and caring for the ecosystems of all animals.

An invocation might be: "Animal Guide, I desire to know and connect with you. Please make yourself known to me so that we may work together."

You can ask for an animal guide to help you with a specific project or aspect of your work, saying, "Animal Spirits, please hear me now as I request support in my work. I desire to connect to an animal guide to support this work for the betterment of all beings and the Earth. Please, may this guide be known to me."

Connect to your animal guide through trance and meditation techniques such as drumming or actively imagining you are traveling to the realm of the animals to meet your animal guide.

Basic Shamanic Concepts of "the Worlds," Animal Spirits, and Connecting to Them

It is generally agreed that there are three main "worlds"—lower, middle, and upper. We and some disembodied beings inhabit this middle world. Angels and higher guides inhabit the upper world, and animal spirits inhabit the lower world. This isn't to say that animals are lesser. They are more in tune with the Earthly plane of consciousness.

Animal spirits are the collective energy of an animal species. They can also include extinct or mythical animals. Your animal guide might have a very distinctive animality (like a personality) when you meet them. They might appear unexpectedly or differently from what the animal looks like in our world. Size, color, and communication ability shift and change in the spirit world. The animal spirit holds a collective frequency and specific traits of those animals. You can find many books and information about animals and what they mean. Rely less on what you are told from the outside and more on what you feel and know internally. In certain cultures, an animal will have specific folklore and mythology around it. Therefore, because of the collective field around that animal, it will often bring through that energy. This doesn't mean you won't receive a different message from a particular animal, so it is up to you to do the work to connect and receive for yourself.

[Practice 34: Connecting to an Animal Guide]

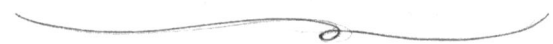

Animal Dance

One of the first offerings with Michelle Hawk was called "Animal Dance." Michelle is an animal shaman, among other things, and has been in deep connection and communication with animal energies her whole life. Besides her healing, channeling, alchemy, and facilitation skills, she is a great DJ. In Animal Dance, we took people on a journey to connect with their animal guide, traveling and studying with it and then embodying it through a merging dance.

Dancing your animal can be a powerful way to connect and learn from your guide. You can invoke their presence, feel them there with you, merge with their energy, and dance their dance. Be sure to disconnect at the end of the dance, thank them, and reflect on their teachings.

[Practice 35: Dancing with Your Animal Guide]

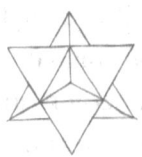

WE ARE AS ONE

Stretching into our skin,

We are One.

In Power,

In presence,

We move through the damp forest.

Eye awakened to your world,

Clear and Purposed.

Hearts beating as one:

Quickening,

Leaping forward,

Reaching,

Finding hold,

Muscles,

Fur,

Tendons,

Claws,

Pulsing,

Stretching,

Owning strength,

Ease of use.

Wisdom of who I am with you infused into my cells,

I hear you calling me,

Feeding me,

Holding me.

As I hold you, we dance this shapeshifter's dance again.

6

ANIMAL, PLANT, MINERAL

I am initiated... by Nature.

Connecting with the energies of animals, plants, and minerals can be beneficial when expanding beyond your internal energy system and field. These relationships enhance your life on many levels and the practices you develop here will benefit you in other connection works.

Initially, you may find it easier to work with these beings than with other types of spirits or the pure energies of the elements— fire, water, air, and earth. Elements are extreme, powerful core essences of energy. Fire can burn, water can drown, air can cause ungroundedness, and even earth energy (the easiest to work with) can create stagnation.

Accessing these Earth-based, living (and I consider minerals living) creatures is easy on your system, fun, and supportive as you dive deeper and develop your abilities. Animals, plants, minerals, and trees give glimpses into archetypal energies living on this planet for a long time. They hold the elements in ways that are gentle to the system. You can easily feel who they are. You know the energy of the skunk, the dog, and the oak tree. They can become powerful allies on the path and further access points to information. They are gateway orders to awaken aspects of yourself to help you heal and grow.

Think of how these things delighted and captivated you as a child. You could spend hours gathering rocks, petting animals, or talking with a tree. Revisiting this childlike perspective helps you rediscover forgotten power and peace. By reconnecting with nature, you better understand your place within the interconnected web of life and enhance your heart-opening appreciation of its profound impact.

The more you allow nature in, the more you appreciate it, feel it, and ache for it. You also feel the pain of nature and humanity's disconnection. It can disturb the senses. But it creates stewardship, empathy, and care for our planet and its inhabitants. As we feel, so might we grow. Allow yourself to experience nature deeply, connect with it, and see how these connections enhance your life and give you power. Find a crystal that "speaks" to you. Allow a favorite animal to "dance" with you. Sit with a plant and meditate with it. Ask them how they would like to serve your life and work and what you can do for them.

In my experience, every being and every place has a song. You will be taught this song only through deep presence, listening, and responding. This is one reason I draw you back to exploration through your voice throughout this text. When you know a being's song, you can sing it to invoke their presence and to bring their medicine into healing.

Notice when a plant, animal, or stone shows up frequently in a period. What is it trying to communicate with you? Becoming quiet and fully present with this being can bring great wisdom and insight. These connections enhance your relationships with the elements. The dolphin teaches about water. The stones and the prairie dogs teach about earth. The phoenix and the snake teach about fire. The eagle teaches about air. By experiencing these elements through these beings, you gain deeper understanding. We are all connected, and the more you embrace and learn from these connections, the more power you gain and the better you can access different energies to support your work.

Element Work

The elements and their corresponding directions and spiritual energies are essential to the healer's life. The more you allow them to work through you, dance through you, and be present with you, the deeper the medicine will be.

During a healing session, you might call in these energies for presence and assistance at the beginning. The deeper work is to be attuned to when these energies should be invoked. With experience, you become familiar with how they like to work through you, and you can utilize them more effectively in sessions.

I am trained and practiced in using the four elements for healing work and the five elements of Chinese medicine. For simplicity, I am offering you the four elements below to correspond to the four directions. I illuminate the five elements in The Healer's Process Practice Manual.

For example:

Fire burns through everything that doesn't serve the highest and best. It is the element of transformation and rapidly shifts things. It can be called upon to heat an area to help energy move, activating what is stagnant or, with its warmth, relaxing held tension. Fire is also helpful as an external portal element that burns away toxic energy that is being pulled out of the system. It supports the lower energy centers, creativity, sexuality, and the heart fire.

Water cleanses and soothes the wounds of the body and soul. It is cooling for inflamed areas. Water holds memory and can be encoded to resonate with energy throughout the body. Water can be used as a portaling element to wash energy out of the area. It supports the kidneys and emotions.

Air purifies and refreshes, removing the old and stale. It brings messages from beyond. It can be used to clear a space quickly. It activates the throat and freedom through expression.

Earth can hold and contain anything that has been released. As the great composter, she receives and transforms all. It provides the stability and structure needed to heal bones and ground those that become too activated energetically. It also supports digestion and a sense of trust and belonging.

This is an ever-evolving process of discovery. Enter into a state of reverence and devotion to these realms. These are the basic tools of the Universe channeled down into the building blocks of the material world. Everything you experience comes from these basic elements. You are made of each and are balanced when you have healthy relationships with them. You can throw yourself off balance by devoting too much attention to one realm. The food you eat, where you live, and the energy practices you do cultivate particular energies in your body, and you must be conscious of your actions in this regard. This is also true for your clients, who usually don't think about these things. By tuning into the elements, you can gather information and use these forces to bring balance and a life in flow.

Elemental frequencies are powerful and real. We didn't New Age these things to life. They have existed long before us and will exist long after. They deserve respect, devotion, and care.

Practices for Connecting to the Elements

It is crucial to establish personal connections with each element. There are many ways to connect with these realms. I encourage you to play, explore, and experiment. Remember, where you put your attention grows and becomes stronger.

It is important to do small actions, rituals, and practices daily and also make time for deeper work. You are forming a relationship with these elements that will last a lifetime. The relationships will change and grow as all do. A heartfelt feeling of devotion is essential. Always open and close your connections with gratitude and thanks.

Fire

Intentionally light a candle, take a moment to connect with the flame, thank it for its service to your life, and sit quietly in meditation while holding a soft gaze on the flickering light. This can be a daily practice to strengthen your relationship. Spend evenings without turning on the lights and do everything by candlelight. This brings a more profound respect for and resonance with the fire element.

Working with fire can be a profound experience. With modern conveniences, we've grown disconnected from the elemental power of fire. Even when camping, one person usually tends the fire, and that might not be you. I encourage you to learn how to light and tend a fire. Knowing how to do so without a lighter or match can be a valuable way to connect with the element of fire. You can easily access instructional videos online or enroll in a survival course to learn this skill.

Ways to Connect to Fire:

- Simply sit and observe the fire. Watch the areas that burn blue, following them as they move. Let your eyes hold a soft gaze as you allow images to emerge from the flames.

- Cook outside on an open flame or even a grill, which will get you close to the heat. Choose spicy foods... hot peppers and blackened meat.

- Learn to spin fire.

- Find a fire walking ceremony. Certain practitioners specialize in this. Please be sure to find a very experienced person. Burns on the feet hurt and can be dangerous.

[Practice 36: Fire Practices]

Water

Water is the lifeblood of this planet. We are comprised mostly of water, and our connection to it is vital. Water has the ability to hold memory. Its molecules are influenced by words, images, thoughts, and prayers. As we sit in a time of environmental degradation and witness the poisoning of our precious waterways, it is crucial that we cultivate a deep, loving relationship with water. Be mindful of how much and how you use this precious resource. While I highly recommend taking baths for their healing and energetic cleansing benefits, be conscious of personal water waste through actions like flushing toilets, running taps, and watering lawns. Be mindful of the foods and products you consume in relation to water usage. Plastics are a major contributor to water pollution and require a significant amount of water to produce. Similarly, animal products, like beef, also require a lot of water. It's worth considering small changes you can make in your daily routine to acknowledge and honor water's role in your life.

Some individuals avoid drinking tap water due to the presence of chemicals, such as fluoride, which can cause calcification of the pineal gland and affect our inner sight. However, there are effective water filters available that can remove these chemicals from tap water. Additionally, some areas have access to natural spring water sources that do not require plastic bottles. Do your research to get the highest quality water available. Purified water lacks vital nutrients, so it's a good idea to add trace minerals to re-mineralize your water before drinking it. This is especially important for supporting your body during healing and channeling works.

Ways to Connect to Water:

- Stop before you drink water and feel a moment of gratitude.

- Eat juicy foods such as melons and other fruits.

- Look into rainwater harvesting and sending greywater to the garden.

- Stand in the rain.

- Make a water mist with light essential oils and regularly spray it on your face.

- Drink more water. As a healer, you'll run a lot of heat through your body in a session, so it is advisable to drink more.

- Charge your water with crystals. Look up which crystals and stones are suitable for charging in water. Some are toxic and should not be placed in water. Others, such as those on the matrix (the hosting stone), will dissolve. They need to be properly cleaned first. They can also be placed inside a test tube in the water so the water doesn't directly contact them. Generally, use rose quartz for heart opening and healing, programmed quartz for different purposes based on your intentions, citrine for collecting solar yang energy, and moonstone or pearl for collecting lunar yin energy.

[Practice 37: Water Practices]

Air

Because air is all around us but unseen, it is the most overlooked element. Strangely, even though our bodies are in constant communion with air as it travels in and out, we rarely think about it unless it is polluted or we are at a high altitude and struggle to breathe.

Notice and acknowledge air regularly. During meditation, bring attention to your breath and feel deep gratitude for the element that sustains you in every moment.

To connect with the air element during meditation, it's best to be in an open area with clean air. You can choose a location where you feel a breeze, which will help you connect with the element. Sitting in a very windy area is not recommended for frequent meditation, as it disperses your energy, so it isn't a sustainable way to cultivate energy. The goal is not necessarily to find a windy place but to fully immerse yourself in the element or energy you're working with. Choose a location that feels right, but avoid smoggy or polluted areas for air meditations. Focus on the sensations of the air moving over your skin. Feel the intermingling of your energy and listen to the messages the air is bringing.

Ways to connect to Air:

- Fly a kite.

- Put up prayer flags.

- Go skydiving, sailing, or flying.

- Put up wind chimes.

- Play with flow flags.

[Practice 38: Air Practices]

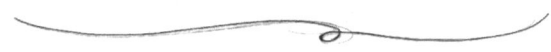

Earth

Earth is the most accessible element to work with. Her large mass provides constant support, supporting you to remain grounded, rooted, and safe. The Earth is a composter for all energies, breaking them into their respective elements. This process helps you manage the energy you release effectively.

Ways to Connect to Earth:

- Eat root vegetables and ancient grains.

- Collect items to make altars or crafts from nature (always ask permission and leave an offering or prayer, acknowledgment for collected objects)

- Place rocks around your home.

- Place your forehead on the ground.

[Practice 39: Earth Practices]

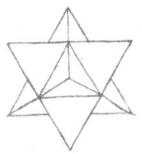

THE ELEMENTS

The wind blew my soul apart.

The fire purified my heart.

The water cleansed my spirit.

Earth held me.

7

MOUNTAIN SHAMAN, RIVER SHAMAN, AND YOUR POWER STONES

*What else do I have but Nature? She supports
and informs every aspect of life.*

hamanism is an Earth-based practice. Those identifying as witches or other healer archetypes also tend to be Earth practitioners. We work with the elements and nature to find power, clarity, and assistance. There is a profound honoring of the Earth and all of her aspects. We walk a path of feeling her deeply and respecting her beings.

When we awaken our inner healer archetypes, we more deeply feel, hear, and know her. We form meaningful relationships with rivers, animals, trees, and minerals. Different individuals are drawn to different places, as this is where their power is sourced. There is a differentiation between a river shaman and a mountain shaman. If you are connected to Mountain Energy, it will call to you. You will have a desire to climb the mountain and sit with it. You will feel fed, nurtured, and held by the mountain. Looking out over the expanse will bring you peace and a feeling of power. You will likely also connect to the trees and animals that find their home there. If you are a river shaman, this is the place you must go to be filled. It is down in the valley, wet and meandering.

Others are filled with power by the ocean, the deep forest of certain trees, the desert, or wetlands. Find your power places and spend as much time there as possible. Consider where you have been drawn since childhood. What natural settings bring you pure joy, and where do you feel your soul being called?

As a child, I was drawn to creeks. I was fascinated by these gentle, life-filled bodies of water. They had a special way of speaking to me. I have found that this is my medicine. During my awakening, I journeyed to Northern California to a forest of redwood trees. A creek bed called to me, and I spent the day there. I had visions, communed with animals, and was spoken to by the creek. She wanted me to be there. She wanted me to take stones when I left to hold the frequency that was a part of my soul. I wasn't looking for stones to take; I was guided to receive them. It was a powerful experience, and I hold these stones to this day to connect to my power source.

We crave nature, and a stone, a branch, or a shell brings joy to the home. We unconsciously strip nature and take from her. We are takers instead of collaborators. Nature wants to work with us and through us. She is the ultimate feminine giver and nurturer. We can easily take from her with little thought.

As we strive to be more conscious, we must align in a reciprocal and honoring relationship with nature. Nature is always willing to provide for us and will draw our attention to what we are meant to take. However, with so many people, we must be mindful of what and how much we take.

I encourage you to gather your power stones from your power place. This process must be infused with prayer and honoring. Listen deeply in these moments. Ask for permission. Ask for forgiveness for any missteps or mistakes you make, and place offerings. These are often food, herbs, or other special items that will not pollute, harm, or alter the environment.

[Practice 40: Power Stones]

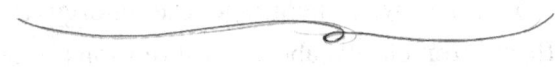

8

DATING YOUR ENERGETICS

This is going to be a beautiful relationship.

One can work with many energies, beings, and guides on this path. It isn't so much about the number of guides you have; it is about the quality of your relationships. Attempting to connect with multiple beings and energies simultaneously can lead to confusion and overwhelm. The work becomes muddied. As you build your Sacred Container, take your time and invite familiar beings. You may have various energies, guides, and angels connecting with you, which can become overwhelming. If you need more clarity regarding their meanings, messages, and roles in your healing work, it is helpful to approach this process like dating.

Your channel might feel like you are sleeping around all over the place. There is nothing wrong with having polyamorous (love with multiple beings) relationships with your energetics, and you will have a council of guides available to you throughout your life. Take time to focus on each relationship individually to nurture them properly.

[Practice 41: Deepening Your Relationship with Your Chosen Guide]

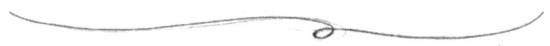

Approach every interaction as you would a cherished romantic partnership. This means being present, consistent, and devotional in your approach. This mindset will encourage the energy to visit frequently and with greater clarity about its intentions and significance in your personal and professional life. By devoting dedicated time to experiencing this energy, you'll be able to recognize its presence in your sessions or daily life and interpret its meaning. Focusing solely on this energy will minimize distractions from other sources.

Creating and maintaining an altar will anchor your frequency and experience together. A working altar is devoted to a specific purpose(s) and is a portal for energy to move into and out of your space. This is a place to sit, make offerings, keep sacred items, pray, and communicate with your guides. When you feel it is time to cycle out of a current altar to focus on working with a different energy, you may want to still maintain an area of honor for this being in your home. If images resonate with this being, do soft gaze open-eye meditation in front of the picture. At the end of connection sessions, always honor the energy and tell them they are free to go but welcome to return when needed.

Through devoted presence and communication (even if it feels one-sided at times) with a being over time, you solidify a relationship that will serve your life and work. At a minimum, your expression of gratitude, admiration, and love will make the world more joy-filled and loving. The potential is that you will gain a powerful ally to call on in times of need or who will actively show up for you when you do your work, offering guidance, support, healing, and protection. You can now invite this being into your Sacred Container.

Depending on the being or energy you are working with, you call that frequency into your life. You will experience changes and shifts based on the energy. Know that some beings, such as Kali, the Hindu Goddess of death and destruction, may shake things up for you as she helps remove anything that isn't serving your higher spiritual path. Working with spiritual beings of high order will almost always bring up your deeper issues, wounds, and inconsistencies. They are being brought to the light to be dealt with, as you have requested, by committing to a spiritual path. The guide offers support and guidance and helps you through the process so you don't have to fear the changes ahead. But you may need to ask for support and help.

9

CLOSING THE SACRED CONTAINER

Too many spiritual people don't know the value
of closing their channel or container.

t may seem helpful to stay open to beings or energies at all times,
but this is not the case. You may notice that spirits come and go
in their ability to produce images or phenomena. This is based
on their ability to sustain themselves in this realm and how much
power they have. Higher-level beings are capable of being present
for extended periods. For others, their life force is insufficient to
sustain them, so they absorb energy from their surroundings. The
energy of psychic people can be siphoned, allowing spirits to take
form and create shifts in the manifest world. This is why psychic
phenomena happen around naturally psychic people. This pulling
of energy isn't intended to be harmful and is not personal. As they
become more entangled, they can eventually deplete your energy
and gradually weaken your field. This is particularly true when
ancestors and family members are summoned to support or observe
the healing process. Closing your channel, intentionally setting your
spiritual boundaries, and living in your sovereignty help you avoid
overly enmeshed spiritual relationships.

Toxic energy released in a session can attract entities through
your portal. They are there to feed off these energies. When you
close the portal you have opened, you prevent attracting the kinds
of beings you would rather not have in your space. This can be
compared to taking out the garbage and putting the lid on the

container to avoid hosting a family of raccoons, bears, or rats.

This information isn't intended to make you fearful or think calling upon your guides and angels is dangerous. Please call upon them and thank them often, and it doesn't always require more effort on your part. But, when opening a portal for healing or channeling, it is important to close the container and seal the space at the end to avoid taking extra risks. Again, come back to the practices you have been learning. Use your physical body to mark the transition with actions such as closing the portal with your hand in a clockwise motion, pulling down the heavens, bowing and acknowledging the directions and energies, thanking and releasing what you have called in, cleansing and purifying the space, and grounding and sourcing yourself to tune into the space and adjust as needed.

[Practice 42: Closing the Sacred Container]

[Practice 43: Closing at the End of the Day]

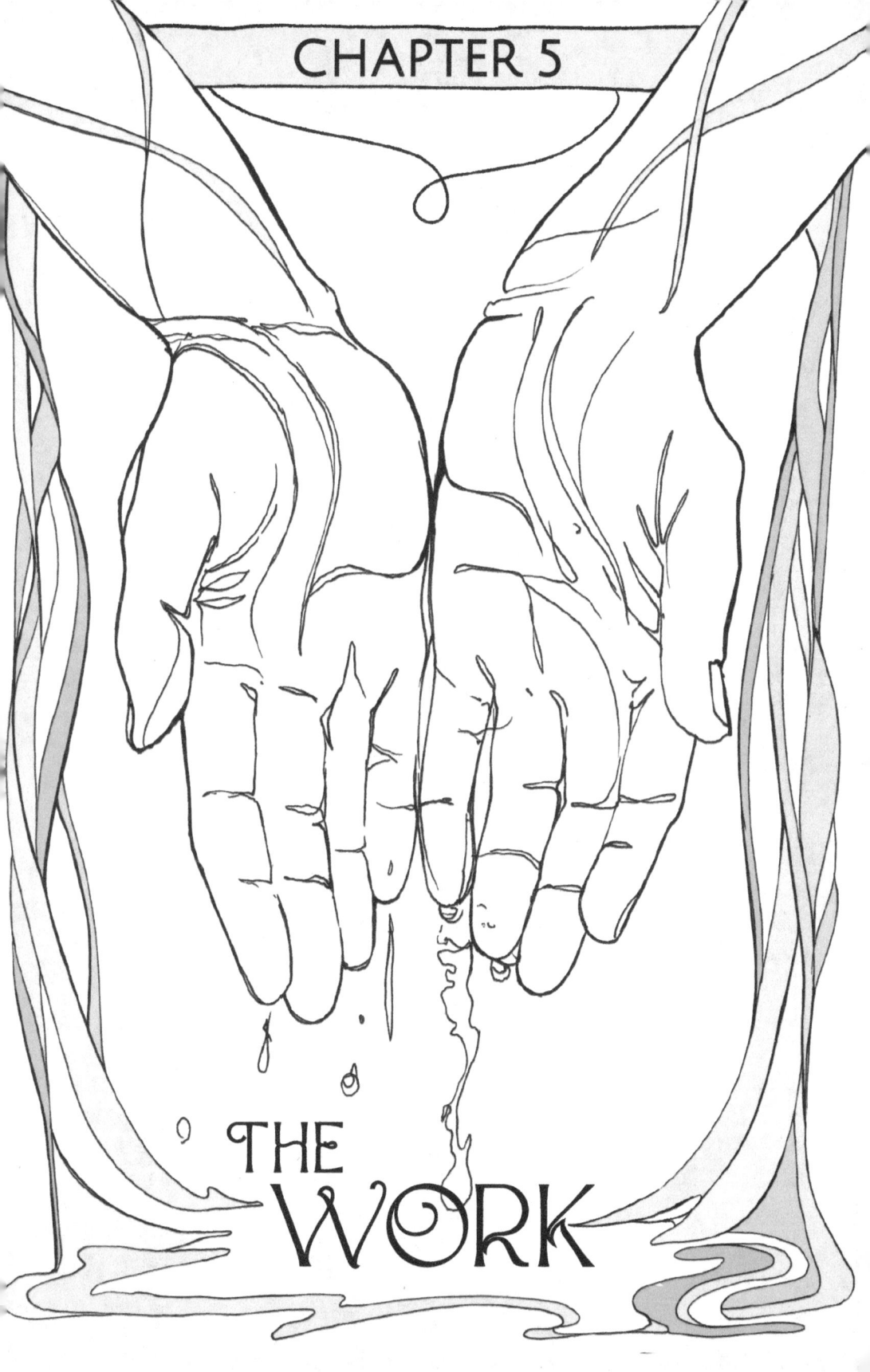

CHAPTER 5

THE
WORK

THE WORK

Your work is the culmination of everything that has come before. It is an interweaving of core soul knowings, the ability to feel and work with your energetic anatomy, and solid relationships with nature and your spiritual team. Your devotion to self-healing, cleansing, and purification in your developing practices offers support and resiliency to step into your authentic way of being.

I use the term 'the work' to mean the work you are designed and trained to accomplish. Don't confuse it with other systems or modalities that discuss 'the work' as a form of self-reflection and inner work.

Throughout this chapter, you will gain deeper insights into how to effectively engage with your clients and support them at a higher level. You will also continue to strip away beliefs and patterns that keep you from inhabiting the unique healer that you are.

The topics in this chapter include:

- Unlocking channeled, shamanic, intuitive healing work.

- Holding space, the assessment process, and working with clients.

- Practicing ethical healing.

- Developing mediumship and channeling.

- Understanding and working with spirits.

- Developing safety and protection in healing and spiritual work.

- Discovering the keys to discernment and avoiding confusion.

- Understanding precision and surrender and when to use them.

- Embracing the unique gifts and aspects of your personal healing work and modality.

1

SHINE YOUR LIGHT

Every healer is unique and deserves to know themselves.

This is where your unique healer shines through. You've begun by focusing on yourself, developing your skills and abilities, building your power and field, and have progressed to working with other energies. You're actively engaging in various healing methods and practices as you allow your authentic self to arise. You have prepared yourself and set the container to confidently enter healing space, trusting yourself to track what is happening and move with the experience as needed.

This chapter delves deeper into being a channel of energy and information, working with different kinds of spirits, and using the structures of the Healer's Process to support your deepest work.

Most of what you have learned happens before or after a client session or in your personal practices. Some parts are revisited or done in session, such as opening the portal and sourcing. You may need a quick cleansing swipe or shake during the session. Naturally, cleansing and purification happen for the client. Calling in guides and setting the container can be done before the session or, depending on your client, while they are in the space.

This section isn't meant to teach you a new modality but rather help you gain access to the healing and information coming through you. This space is often overlooked in demonstrations of modalities, particularly those focused on physical healing or coaching methods that rely on scripts and focus on the mental. I encourage you to stretch the limits of what you do and find your edges. Even seasoned practitioners often want to do or say something in a session and hold themselves back, fearing it might seem weird. In truth, the gold often lies in the moments when you feel compelled to speak a particular phrase, touch a specific spot, make a sound, add a crystal, wave, or clap your hands. These actions may tap into something profound and have a significant impact. Most people appreciate authentic work. They are crying out for it. This person trusts you. Trust yourself.

That said, being mindful of your client's spiritual and energetic viewpoints is important. Introduce new concepts gradually as you feel their openness. People can shut down if their worldview is pushed too far too fast. Calling in guides or beings they can't relate to or have no concept of might cause them to put up defenses. Remember, your intention is the key; you can do much of this work silently. If you feel a call to welcome energy, you don't have to state it aloud. Knowing your client's belief systems can help determine what's appropriate and beneficial. Being consistent with their cosmology of energies, guides, saints, or religious figures is helpful as they relate to and trust those beings. If someone is a Christian, they might appreciate Jesus or the Virgin Mary, but if a strict Christian upbringing abused them, naming those beings might shut them down. Know your clients enough to understand how to open them with your invocations, or don't include this work out loud. Ask questions, be curious, honor, and respect who they are and where they came from. Sometimes, less is just right, as many people are okay with energy concepts but not spirits.

The Deeper Truth of Your Work

When I defined my healing work as structural bodywork, I struggled to keep to myself the sounds and phrases that naturally arose during sessions. My innate healing abilities urged me to express myself through speaking in tongues or light language, singing tones into people's bodies, and moving energy in ways I had never seen demonstrated before. Although my guides told me to be seen as I am for years, I kept my true, channeled work bottled up. My body put an end to my hiding. I developed severe swelling in my joints, tendonitis, and pain throughout my body until I started sharing the deeper truths of my work and stuck with who I am in session and the things I am most called to do and teach. When I let my intuitive expressions out, people had profound sessions. The songs and strange things helped people. Over time, I stopped minimizing these parts of my work and let them take up the space they needed to evolve. My body healed, I developed trust in my work, and I learned how to love the parts of myself that I had labeled as weird and too much.

A part of my consciousness has loudly questioned my actions in sessions or healing events. Even amid something that felt aligned and right, a voice said, "What are you doing? Are you crazy?" There have also been instances where I felt remorseful about what tumbled out of my mouth during a profound state of presence. Sometimes, I have spoken in a direct and forceful manner and then felt shocked and a bit ashamed for speaking so bluntly. These were often the most impactful moments, and the feedback I received was that these words or actions were responsible for creating massive shifts and healing. Over time, I stopped second-guessing myself (even when that inner voice shows up). This will happen for you, too, if you give yourself permission to speak and do the things you can't explain. It is a practice of surrender. You have to, at some point, accept your abilities. You might even have to accept that you are magic. This may be the greatest gift you give yourself and the world.

2

HOLDING SPACE

*And the space she held was impeccable. So much
so that there was nothing more to do.*

Even though "holding space" is an amorphous term, I'm sure you've had the experience of feeling held by someone. In the space of active listening and presence, you could open up and reveal yourself. Being witnessed created an internal shift, and your struggles seemed lighter. Clarity emerged, and calm-centeredness was possible even though circumstances remained the same.

Our deep presence is a state of being rather than something we try to do. Unfortunately, this crucial aspect of healing work can be overlooked or undervalued because it isn't the "modality" people pay for when they sign up for a session.

Sometimes, we inadvertently rush critical moments to focus on the specific techniques they are paying for. This can be particularly true if we are accustomed to providing hands-on healing work on a table. I've had to learn the balance between being present and attentive and actively engaging in the work. As the focus of my sessions shifted towards listening, reflecting, holding space, and teaching rather than solely providing healing work, I initially felt uneasy. I worried that my clients might feel shortchanged if I did not physically touch them or if we did not accomplish enough. However, despite my concerns, many clients said these were the best sessions.

Many people live without anyone to confide in about their true experiences. They lack space-holding, supportive relationships. During spiritual and energetic awakenings, individuals need to share their experiences and receive validation that they are not crazy and are not alone in this journey. Instead, they are experiencing something normal with a recognizable process. Many people express that one of the most valuable spaces I hold is that they can share their experiences without being judged or receiving a blank response, which they might receive from someone they know. Those in upper-level management, entrepreneurs, spiritual leaders, advisors, healers, and others who provide support to others often lack adequate support for themselves. Everyone experiences pain, grief, and life changes that require reflection.

We have a human need to be seen and supported. The healing relationship, no matter what kind, affords people this opportunity. How you hold space and show up in sessions can and will change as you develop a deeper presence and the ability to trust your intuitive work. When you are holding space for someone, to them, it feels effortless. The sensation is magical because it heals and transforms without being forceful.

Again, your intention is the key here. The highest intention is that wholeness and health already exist. This opens up potentiality fields as you see them in a way that they have not been able to see themselves. This reflection, even from a silent, internal place, vibrates throughout your field and affects theirs. You are present with a possibility they have yet to discover. It anchors within the collective field and has a greater potential to emerge.

At these moments, open and surrender to what most needs to come through. Listening, questions, and reflection allow clients to find their own answers. When someone has been fully seen and moves through powerful, previously suppressed emotions, it creates space for healing to occur. The surface issues of the day peel back to reveal yesterday's core wounds and emotions that have become trapped in the body and field. Working with these deeper issues, there is the ability to make space for a new way of being as adjustments to their energy, physical body, or perspective create the shifts needed to move forward.

Be Soft and Flexible

In this emergent work, you can have a plan but be open to flexibility. Provide your clients with an experience encompassing openness, vulnerability, calm presence, and purity of intention. Once their nervous system can attune to these qualities, they will embody them. These are the missing elements that affect all their relationships. By giving them a resonant frequency to tune into, they will feel safe enough to trust it within themselves.

You are helping to clear the plague of not-enoughness. People translate "I'm not enough" into their healing process. By providing a safe space for them to be heard and guiding them through their emotions, you help them find healing and relief. This requires a level of patience that isn't commonplace in modern society. Since childhood, we have been rushed and expected to keep up with others. When we couldn't, we may have been shamed. Patience acts as a soothing balm. When they aren't pressured to perform perfectly, recover quickly, or move on hastily from grief and pain, they can relax and unwind from the trauma of never being good enough.

Surrender into the truth that whatever your client needs for their highest and best will happen. This could mean that your sessions have more open space. It may require doing less and being quiet more. Silence can be uncomfortable between people. Many can handle this no more than they can take sitting in silence by themselves. Sometimes, people try to cope with emptiness by seeking constant stimulation, talking, or noise. Considering the impact of meditation, which involves sitting in silence and being present, embracing silence can also benefit session work. New possibilities can arise by waiting and observing instead of rushing to solve a problem or fill a void.

Being fully present and open to all possibilities is a humble way of being. Instead of focusing on trying and doing, take the time to discover your own beingness. Step aside and allow guidance from higher forces to come through. This will help push intellectualizing out of the way and create space for higher knowledge to emerge.

3

ETHICS IN PRACTICE

Integrity is transformational.

Being a healer is a tricky business. There is no governing board to establish specific guidelines for our behavior. We are not held accountable by licensing, and healing work is largely unregulated, much like coaching. Unfortunately, the field is open to unscrupulous individuals who exploit vulnerable people and many who do not adhere to ethical standards in this line of work. It is essential to contemplate your ethical standards and revisit them regularly. Please consider that your teachers, healers, and trainers may not practice ethically. You may have seen it demonstrated that certain ethical standards are not essential to care. Remember that someone can be highly educated and skilled and still have aspects of their work that harm their client or community.

When clients are treated energetically, they open and enter an altered state of consciousness. Their external boundaries become relaxed or disappear. They are inherently vulnerable in the healing relationship. It is crucial to maintain professional boundaries and standards as outlined below:

Expectations

You must be aware of your client's expectations of the work you will undertake together. It is crucial to have clear and honest communication about the process and possible outcomes. It's not necessary to make grand promises to attract clients. Some business coaches may suggest this, but avoid making unrealistic, exaggerated, or untrue statements. Making promises that can't be fulfilled will only make you feel stressed, nervous, and overwhelmed. It can leave the client distrusting healers and healing, creating roadblocks to further development. Any agreements that you make should be honored. This includes the timing of sessions, payment schedules, payment amounts, follow-up procedures, and delivery of products and services.

Scope of Practice

Sometimes, a client will present with an issue that you're not familiar with, trained in, or comfortable enough to work with. This could be a mental health condition or a medical diagnosis that falls outside your area of expertise. Maybe someone is pregnant or injured, and you are unsure if your work is safe for them. Your modality may be contraindicated for this person. This is why having intake forms and conversations with people is helpful before beginning your work. These should cover mental, emotional, and physical issues and past diagnoses. You should know what medications your client is taking to avoid recommending something that could be harmful. Numerous medications can interact with plant medicines, herbs, and certain foods. If you aren't sure about something someone tells you or puts on a form, ask. Research when you don't know something, and don't go blind into situations.

I recommend having a list of other practitioners to refer clients to when needed. You can even create mutually supportive referral systems. You aren't supposed to know everything or work with every person. Cancer patients, pregnant people, children, older individuals, and those with mental health issues are all highly specialized and specific population segments. They require special care in some modalities. If you are starting out, you aren't expected to offer exorcisms and other advanced techniques without those pieces of training. You can assist many people, but for those who require specific expertise, it is best to refer them to someone else.

If someone contacts you about work you don't want to do, there is nothing wrong with referring them to someone else. I rarely work with severely sick or terminal patients. This isn't to say I never do this work, but I typically refer them to healers who specialize in these populations. If you cannot accept someone's lifestyle or choices because of your viewpoints or beliefs, send them to a practitioner aligned with their values. It is highly damaging when someone seeks support and the person they see doesn't believe in or actively criticizes or undermines their right to personal, sexual, or gender expression or orientation. If your religious beliefs are fundamental to your work, be clear and upfront about that in your marketing materials. You also may not be the best practitioner due to culture, ethnicity, gender, background, or presentation. You may actively trigger someone through your presence, no matter how educated, open, or accepting. Be aware of the societal challenges that different groups face, educate yourself, and know that even with good intentions and education, you might not be the best choice for someone. This may require an uncomfortable conversation to determine if the healing relationship aligns with the client's needs.

You may worry that turning down potential clients could lead to failure, especially when income is needed. However, not everyone is your client, and you aren't the practitioner for everyone. Being a part of the flow that refers someone to a practitioner who can genuinely help them will serve your business's energy in the long term. Having a client that you cannot help is frustrating for everyone involved. Ensure success for you and the client by directing them to where they can receive proper support.

Consent

It is essential to obtain informed consent in your work. This involves ensuring that the client is fully aware of your work and has given their consent, preferably in writing. It is also important to ask for consent before initiating physical contact at the beginning of a session. This allows them to voice their yes and know they are in control and respected. Consider asking for consent before touching other areas of the body, especially with a new or nervous client.

If you do work involving the genitals or sexual area in any way, the person must give full consent before any work can be done. This means before they have been engaged physically or energetically at all. Once someone is relaxed or in a trance, it is too easy to say yes when they mean no. They can also drop out of their bodies and allow things to be done that they will regret or feel traumatized by later. There is an inherent power imbalance in the healing relationship. There is an even more significant imbalance once someone is vulnerable on a treatment table. Be clear before the session about what might happen, and don't go beyond that. You might get a message or intuitive awareness in a session that someone needs sexual healing work. That is excellent information, but it should never be acted on in that session if it was not fully agreed upon beforehand. If deeper or further work needs to be done, it can be discussed later to occur in a different session. Many healers make big mistakes here. This can affect your business, brand, and reputation and create legal issues, and it is a gross violation of spiritual law to go against someone's will in a healing session. You will carry this with you even if no one finds out.

Sex and Relationships

Healing is emotionally vulnerable and highly energetic. The person treating or the client can lose objectivity and transfer sexual feelings to the other. It can be highly damaging for sexual energy or touch to enter a healing session. Sexual healing work is only to be done by those specifically and thoroughly trained in these modalities. Those who specialize in sexual healing should receive training in the ethical standards of their practice. Far too often, those seeking sexual healing are further traumatized by practitioners who put their desires or ego over the needs of their clients.

Don't act sexually or romantically toward your client. One or both of you may have feelings emerge. Acting on those feelings or accepting advances can harm the healing process. It feels unethical for me to engage romantically or sexually with a client even after the healing relationship is complete. But I know this happens. Situations arise, and it doesn't serve you to be blind to the possibility of this. If you feel this person might be a significant connection, stop treating them and give yourself time to clear the energy of the previous dynamic to honor everyone involved. If it is meant to be, it will still be meant to be months from now. There are also different depths of healing relationships. You might feel different rules apply between someone who once came to a large group workshop and someone under personal therapeutic care. You should have a pre-determined and outlined standard if this issue arises. Be aware that people talk, and being known as someone who connects intimately with clients or students will bring your integrity as a practitioner into question.

The focus placed on boundaries in Chapter 2, Building the Field, will support you in knowing, stating, and keeping clear boundaries and holding them for clients. Clients can easily mistake the energy and feelings they get from session work to mean they are in love or lust with their practitioner. It is up to you to hold the container and keep your clients safe. It is easy to manipulate energy into feelings. Explore your unconscious desires and motivations and consider the potential harm to your client, you, and your entire community. Others receiving benefits could choose to leave your care because of what they see as unethical behavior. This could have a long-term impact on their ability to trust new practitioners.

Confidentiality

Keep all information and details of your clients confidential. This ensures trust and safety. There are some times when this can be broken to report an incident to the appropriate authority:

- When a client is a danger to themselves (suicide) or others (homicide).

- In case of a life-threatening emergency.

- In the case of child or elder abuse.

- There may be grey areas that you are unsure of, such as domestic violence issues between adults. You can look to professional standards for therapists, but they vary by state on this reporting requirement. Helping someone navigate a situation and create a plan to stay safe may be the priority. The possibility of abuse, addiction, or other personal crises arising during your work with someone is another reason it is valuable to have a mentor and awareness of different types of practitioners and organizations to refer people. If you are out of your depths, a social worker, therapist, crisis or rehabilitation center may be able to offer support. Learn when to pull in these resources and how to find them.

Assessment

Although often overlooked, the assessment process is illuminating as it uncovers information that might not come up during appointments. Practitioners avoid proper assessments because they don't want to use session time for this process—an online assessment form filled out before the first session solves this problem.

This form should request information from their physical, energetic, mental, emotional, and spiritual aspects. Physical signs and symptoms can inform energetic issues—emotional and spiritual pain cause symptoms in the body. Everything is interconnected, and healing is a holistic journey that requires peering into all parts of the self. A good assessment will allow your clients to self-reflect and get honest about all aspects of their lives, as they often come with a particular focus and may not see the layers of issues at play. Over time, you will build your assessment process based on your work.

Here are some examples of important topics to discuss:

Physical: Illnesses, surgeries, pain, medications, supplements, dietary habits and cravings, digestive issues and bowel movements, physical activity, and exercise.

Energetic: Energy levels, sleep patterns, awareness of energy and stress levels, and how they approach social situations.

Mental: Connection to short—and long-term memory (this will give information about possible repressed memories, trauma, and current health), thought patterns such as ruminating thoughts, beliefs about self and the world, and satisfaction with life. Past or current mental health issues and treatments. You can also address the expectations of working together here.

Emotional: The ability to love self and others, relationship satisfaction, emotional patterns, and the ability to deal with challenging emotions.

Spiritual: Connection to God, Source, etc., spiritual or meditation practices, meaning, purpose, ability to follow their path, and experiences with non-ordinary states of reality.

In all of this, you are getting an idea of:

- If they have a supportive home and work environment.

- Their current state on all levels, as well as desires, goals, and needs.

- Self-care practices and the ability to integrate your work.

- What might come up in your sessions and work together, as well as a treatment plan.

- This informs session work, homework, and further support they might need.

JOURNAL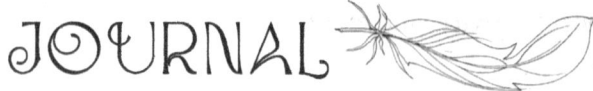

Craft your ethical standards. Explore the principles behind your commitments of conduct. These can include standards of actions you will refrain from and those you are committed to upholding. Often, those you commit to uphold are anchored in your values, such as compassion, fairness, and honesty. Consider anything and everything that might come up in your work and how you declare you will handle issues.

4

HELPING THEM HELP
THEMSELVES

Belief creates healing. Words create belief.

Healing depends on trust and belief. If someone lacks faith in you, your healing method, or themselves, healing can be more challenging. This explains why one person may require longer to heal from the same issue than others and why some people are a breeze to work with while it's like chipping at a stone block with others.

Healing can be a slow process, as building trust takes time. People come from broken homes and traumatic situations and struggle to trust others and themselves. The healing process happens when someone opens up and allows themselves to heal. They heal themselves within the sacred container you create. They trust the container because they trust you. You are calm, sourcing yourself, not wanting or needing anything from them, and have a presence of patient kindness, respect, and availability. You are confident in your ability to hold them in their darkest places and most challenging moments. They are safe to have an experience in your presence, so their guard drops, and they are open to the work.

Watch Your Words

Your most powerful healing instrument is your voice as you utilize prayers, songs, and invocations to bring in powerful energies. Your words vibrationally affect the space you're in, yourself, and whoever else is present. Enunciation, exploration of vowels and consonants, vocal tone, and inflection significantly impact your chosen words. They can have a hypnotizing effect on the client, who falls into a more receptive trance-like state. Repetition is a powerful form of incanting invocations. I have included this in some of the earlier prompts. For example: "I call, I call, I call. Welcome, welcome, welcome. Thank you, thank you, thank you, thank you."

Consider this when calling in spiritual help through invocations, giving people suggestions, guiding them, and bringing them back to their bodies at the end of the session. With every word, you have the power to deepen their experience.

When engaging in healing work, be mindful of the messages you convey. The mind and beliefs are powerful forces. As you recognize the power dynamics inherent in the healing relationship, understand that your words can have lasting impacts on a person's life. What you communicate is what people internalize. This is wonderful because you can offer people fresh perspectives and help them see themselves in a new light. Your insights inspire them to fly to new heights. However, people can fixate on something a practitioner tells them and use it to stay stuck. If we inform someone of their predetermined nature, destiny, or future prospects, we may deprive them of their autonomy, options, and exploration. We may see only one perspective, opportunity, or potentiality. It might be precisely what is needed to assist in the healing, or it might be unnecessary.

This is one reason I shifted my work over the years toward guiding my clients to do their own journey work. I help them explore their body, psyche, and other realms, but what they discover is up to them. I then support deeper work with what is illuminated. I check in more with my guides and higher self if I need to share what I receive and practice a level of discernment many practitioners lack. I receive a lot of information, but I always ask if sharing is of the highest service or might keep them stuck. I prefer to lead people to their own answers and work in the direction they are called instead of forcing them toward what I see. I work energetically on what I see and offer homework and practices to support that. Still, it isn't always necessary to talk about what I am aware of because it can become one more story that the person becomes wrapped up in, and through our work together, I want them to be free of so many stories.

Natural Conclusions

Allow your clients to come to their own conclusions when possible. Ask questions instead of giving a diagnosis. Peeling the layers off of stigmatized diagnosis is a process. What you say could become an overwhelming truth and mantra for your client. I have heard so many times, "I went to this doctor, psychic, healer, astrologer... and she said this . . . " And that is how they live their lives.

Often, doctors diagnose an illness, and the person lives into the illness. If they are told they have a certain amount of time to live, they will hold that as truth. There have been cases of mixed-up lab tests sending a healthy person down a declining path toward death, and a sick person told they are healthy, eventually having no sign of illness. They can become as stuck in what you give them as a diagnosis from a doctor. If you tell someone that they are broken, sick, or flawed in a particular way, they can take that to mean that this is how they are, and that is it. They might hold it so tightly that they become more of that instead of using it as a pivot point to change. People stuck in a victim mindset can take the information they collect from practitioners and use it to feed that mindset and make themselves sicker.

This is a fine line for healers, psychics, and coaches. Sometimes, it is easier to tell someone what you see and know and how to fix their problems. But are you creating a dynamic where the person is dependent, stuck, and unsure of themselves? How can you help people to own themselves, their path, and their voice through their process as you empower them to know that they are healing themselves?

Be willing to ask yourself if you are sharing from a sense of being not enough and wanting to give more. Remember that intuitive and psychic information is one lens of possibility. It may be one timeline of truth. Not everything you see or know needs to come out of your mouth. Do you know this client well enough to know how they will take it and what they will do with it? Can you offer a path forward, or are you putting something out there that will lead them into despair, which isn't helpful for healing?

You follow your intuition as a channel and allow messages and information to come through. Still, there is a further refining of these gifts, a deeper precision that can be cultivated by questioning the highest service you can offer each individual in every moment. This is being an empowering practitioner. Is there a risk that they will no longer need us? I hope so.

5

TODAY ISN'T A GOOD
DAY TO BE A SHAMAN

Healing is a collaboration sport.

Some of the best advice I've received from a mentor was that if you can't be fully present and in your power, don't do the session. You put yourself and your client at risk. Never be afraid to cancel a session. In such cases, saying, "I want to give you the best possible experience. Can we reschedule?" is better.

As helpers and healers, we don't want to let people down. We know they are in crisis or pain, and we want to serve them. We let old stories of worth sneak in, "Will they be disappointed in me? Will they not come back? Will I let them down?"

People are kinder, more flexible, and more accommodating than we think. Often, when I don't feel like doing a session, something is coming up in their life, too, and it works out for the best. At other times, the core thing we need to work on will be better addressed later. Shifts in the surrounding energetics are also at play, and changes in the moon or stars might help the work more later.

The more I worked with psychics and intuitives, the more likely it would be that I would get a message from a client session saying, "I am not sure why, but it feels like we aren't supposed to work today." This was always when I was sitting and thinking about rescheduling the session due to something coming up. The people we work with can read energy, even if they don't consider themselves intuitive. This is another reason to be impeccable in your self-care and honest with what you are capable of taking on at any given time.

Most of the time, your practices will help you shift quickly as you clear, ground, source, and get to a good place for your work. In your commitment to working toward the highest for your client, you must also consider you're human. Take care of yourself. This is deep listening at every level of being and asking yourself and your guides, "Is this a good time to work?" If you are overly tired, sick, or depleted, you run a risk of taking on others' energy when you go ahead with a session. Emotionally intense experiences need your attention instead of trying to shift focus quickly to your work. It is also advisable to pay attention if you're overly hungry, too full, or dehydrated before a session. And, of course, you should not work if you have been under the influence of alcohol or substances.

Some practitioners find it valuable to map out energy patterns to determine the best times to work for them. This means journaling to determine when you have more energy and when you need to take breaks during the day. It is also helpful to track your monthly cycle of energy. This will be affected by your hormonal cycle. When you are aware of this, you can schedule your time for the greatest effect. Societal conditioning tries to make us all the same. It is better to know yourself and create the conditions for the best possible experience for everyone involved.

6

UNLOCKING MEDIUMSHIP

At a certain point, she couldn't deny her magic any longer.

The fact you found your way to these pages shows you are inclined toward the magical and mystical—there is even more of you waiting to emerge. I am offering many tools and ways of approaching your work, but more than anything, I want you to trust yourself to be open to complete authenticity.

Humans have an inherent inclination towards spirituality and a desire to connect with higher realms. Our very being is attuned to the flow of energy, and we strive to gain greater insight by tapping into the Divine. We are undergoing a global evolution that will transform our species in ways we can hardly imagine. We are all part of this awakening and are actively involved in this revolution, paving the way for a brighter future.

As ambassadors and change agents, we pull through wisdom, guidance, and support from other realms. We are aware of a collective shift that requires an energetic and emotional re-patterning. We are here to do the heavy lifting, and it requires us to step into the fullness of who we are, no matter how odd or scary that might be for each one.

We are the mediums by which the change is happening. No wonder so many are called to the realms of mediumship in some form or another.

Mediumship is a natural human phenomenon. It is a bridge between two or more things, planes, densities, and times. It is being a receptive vessel carrying from the spiritual to the mundane, usually through the process of energy to thought forms to words and actions. In essence, it is the role of the messenger and the medium through which power, information, healing, and guidance can emerge. In our culture, mediumship is often ascribed primarily to talking to the dead. This is but one aspect of mediumship, which is communication and translation with any spiritual force. Forms of mediumship include:

- Clairvoyance: Clear Seeing

- Clairaudience: Clear Hearing

- Clairsentience: Clear Feeling: Past, Present, Future, Emotional State, Places

- Claircognizance: Clear Knowing

- Clairalience: Clear Smelling

- Clairgustance: Clear Tasting

- Psychometry: Picking information up from objects

- Healing Work: Working with Doctor Spirits and spiritual energy

- Medium of Psychophony: Conscious or unconscious trance channeling

- Psychography: Channeled writing

As healers, we utilize many of these skills in our sessions. Although channeling is one form of mediumship, I will discuss it here and use the terms mediumship and channeling interchangeably. In this context, you will see that being a medium or a channel is being open and sensitive enough to allow healing or other information to move through you. It is also being grounded, sourced, and stable enough not to be shaken off balance by its occurrence in your life and work. It is the skill of learning how to translate.

You might think, "Nah, that isn't me; I'm not a channel," your clients will be even less likely to consider this possibility. You might not think you are a medium, but you still experience untrained, accidental forms of mediumship that can cause confusion, energy leaks, or fear. Here are some signs of a natural predisposition to being a medium:

- Interest in the spirit realms

- Psychic abilities and knowing

- Subtle, seeing things out of the corners of the eyes

- Strange movements and sounds when meditating

- Strongly affected by places and objects

- Profuse writer or artist

- Feel something that you make or do is better or more genius than your actual ability

- Family connection (look especially at grandparents)

- Friends say, "You always have the best answers and feedback."

- Drop into the flow state easily

To advance as a medium, you must understand, train, and practice. Much of this involves getting past your blocks, fears, beliefs, and doubts.

Do You Deny Who You Are?

We avoid being a medium or doing intuitive, channeled healing in many ways. Often, it is simply because we don't know any better. When we take on a body, we forget our eternal soul and connection to the unseen world. What we do remember is systematically taken from us. We are taught that to believe in science, we must not believe in anything spiritual or mystical. To believe in religion, we must distance ourselves from our intuitive awareness and personal power. We are taught to fear the unseen and live by strict rules dictated by both religious and secular leaders.

Others don't want to deal with being "this" in the world because "this" is weird and outside the norm. As you have seen in the study of the archetypes, there are gifts and shadows to having spiritual, energetic, and intuitive abilities. To hold this role in society, we are automatically set apart. Being excluded feels unsafe as we are evolutionarily wired to stay within the embrace of family and community. The internal drive to remain safe through belonging can keep us small and unexpressed. We might then create many strategies to repress our natural abilities and inclinations. Over time, they are solidified into unconscious habits. Let's look at a few ways that we deny our channel.

- Busy, Busy, Busy. Filling calendars, rushing from one thing to another, and taking care of everyone and everything else.

- Avoiding being alone and quiet.

- Focus on left-brain activities. Do you pride yourself on your intellect and ability to figure things out? Do you discount intuitive hits? After work, do you continue to engage in more left-brain activity? Do you allow for creative and non-linear pursuits?

- Denial. Do you discount when synchronicity occurs? Do you brush off messages? Do you have disdain or even feel repulsed by spiritual people? Do you avoid spiritual practices?

- Avoiding supportive relationships. Do you only hang out with people who would think this is too weird and woo-woo?

- Engaging in self-medication and addictions that keep you numb and turned off. This includes things like food and media.

- Doubt. There is such a thing as healthy doubt, which is a part of discernment. In this form, you are still open to all possibilities but are curious and ask questions about your experience or who you are communicating with. There is another form of doubt which actively rejects receiving. This is the initial doubt of all spiritual experiences as real and immediately denying when something non-ordinary occurs. If the initial response to every experience is doubt, that doesn't give you anywhere to go. You might hear a voice in your head saying, "Is this real?" all the time. You can speak to that voice and ask that it step back and give you space to experience before you immediately shut down your connections.

- Fear. You were taught to fear the unseen realms. Think of every horror movie that has reinforced that contact with the unseen will end in death or worse. Fear is natural and common, but spinning in fear is highly unhelpful. If you have fear, that is fine. What do you need to do to acknowledge it and move through it?

JOURNAL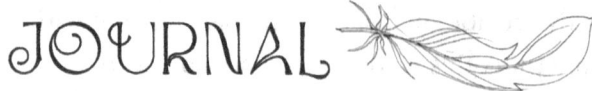

Go through the list above, and for each, self-reflect and write about what you notice. Don't just glance at the sentence. Breathe, be present with where it might be true. Here are some things to consider:

- Where do you see this, or where have you seen this in the past?

- Where did you learn this?

- How could these avoidance practices be trying to keep you safe?

- What steps could you take to address this?

7

BEING THE CHANNEL

I am a channel. As are you.

hen I started channeling, I had no idea what I was doing. I had a massive mystical awakening without guidance. My channel opened spontaneously. I didn't try to become a channel. It simply is what I am. Maybe this has been your experience. The shock of this type of awakening can cause you to shut down. It can also feel impossible to shut down, which is scary and confusing.

If you had access to these experiences in the past but pushed them away, you can reactivate your gifts. Even if you only remember a glimmer of childhood experiences, they are still a part of you. They may need time to find their full awakening. Through practice, these gifts will become skills. Start with the intention to reopen this aspect of yourself.

What if you feel like you have never had these abilities or gifts? That's okay. These skills can be learned. They are a part of being human. It is more normal than you think. Again, your intention is critical. You are in charge. Request what you want from the Universe and open yourself to embody this reality. The clearer you are, the more easily you will integrate into the being you're designed to be in this lifetime. Your work to address your archetypal and inner child wounds, cleanse and purify your system, and work with your sacred container will enable you to do this more easily.

[Practice 44: Opening and Closing the Channel]

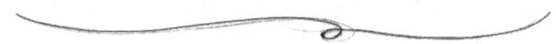

Protection

Remember, a legion of beings of light hold you. You still have to ask for assistance, guidance, and protection. Call on your guardian angels, power animals, and personal guides. Ask for Archangel Michael or other protective forces when you need help. Invoke the highest Divine Light and Love to be present with you.

For example:

- "I call upon you, Archangel Michael, to bathe me in your blue light of protection as I go about my work today."

- "I call upon my guardian angels and the beings of light that support me to hold me in a bubble of protective light."

- "I call up on my animal guide, ..., to be with me as I travel into the unseen realms. Protect and guide me."

The real secret here is to be that energy. Be the energy of a powerful guardian angel from the inside out. You are missing the point if you are coming from fear and the need to be saved. As much as possible, focus on protecting your own energy from collapsing or becoming distracted. This means you are aware of your energy, thoughts, and feelings and choosing to actively work with them. Protection isn't coming from outside of you. It is you. Come from your highest self, your ultimate spiritual connection, full of light and love, radiating. When we aren't radiating is when we feel that we need protection. It is good to call upon light and protection, but realize you are calling this up within you to embody and radiate outward. This is why the inner radiance practices of cultivating energy in the belly, building the core of light through the center of the body, and radiating to build the fields are vital to this kind of work.

What Does Being a Channel Feel Like?

Being a channel of healing and information feels and manifests differently for people. Explore and be curious. It might not look or sound like you want. In fact, it might be weird or even silly. I have experienced and seen others have odd shaking, tics, grotesque faces, uncontrollable limbs, and profuse sweating. People say that I sometimes sound like an old Romanian lady.

It isn't easy to describe the experience of the channel, but the feeling I get in this state is a mixed balance of being very present and aware, yet as if I have stepped back. It is as if I am sitting in the back of my brain. The experience of surrender is needed for the channel to open. I relax and engage my yin eyes, which are soft, open, and receptive. This helps me enter the space that I need to get to for the information to come through. Although I may have my eyes open, I do not fully see everything in the environment. I ask for a different sight to emerge. Things are blurry, with colors or images floating through my consciousness as I am drawn to areas of the body that need healing. Instead of looking directly into someone's eyes as I would in conversation, I accept that looking up and away helps me receive more easily. I also know that certain information streams from particular guides inhabit different zones around my body. I know that looking up and to the right gives me better access to one specific guide while leaning back and feeling behind me to the right helps me access another.

Time and space fall away. I have difficulty processing numbers, writing, telling time, and other left-brain activities. It sometimes seems like a journey to get back to the real world. Over time, this has become easier. The structure of the Healer's Process allows for entering into this timeless space. Through repetition in your personal healing and channeling sessions for yourself, you begin subconsciously tracking the larger structure you are moving through. You can be open to what is emergent because you are confident in your ability to cleanse, purify, ground, and receive support. Knowing and embodying the structure allows your truest flow and channeled state to emerge and be safe and effective.

The longer I do this work, the more I am initiated into its ability. For a while, I could only speak in tongues/ light language (more on this later) when I was channeling certain information. It took a lot of energy to translate what I was saying. I often knew what I was saying, yet getting it into English was an incredible struggle. My brain felt tired from the experience. I have now been offered the ability to translate messages most of the time. When I can't, I realize this person does not need English. This is part of the transmission.

Now, I can look up and bring through a message in the middle of a conversation. In the past, this kind of split focus took more work. My path to embodying who I am as a channel has been a process of consistent practice and releasing judgments of myself.

Anatomy of the Channel

Your physical and energetic bodies are highly involved in channeling. Your bodies will change, and often quite rapidly, from engaging in this work. Moving these energies and connecting to spiritual forces creates shifts in vibration and spontaneous healing, often requiring a massive purge of stagnant energy and trauma. This can create pain, exhaustion, and even symptoms of illness. This doesn't mean you are doing it wrong. It means you are going through your own personal healing and balancing process instigated by your work. From here, you must determine how to best care for yourself. Even projecting energy in a healing session requires you to be fully sourced and creates heat in the body, which dehydrates. This will often mean a need for more water, food, rest, and alone time.

Your requirements may change dramatically. You might need two to three more hours of sleep a night. You might need to change your diet drastically. You may feel called to change your relationship to eating animal products, either consuming less or more. I am not here to dictate to someone what they should do, and this is often a decision based on deep, personal ethics. You might dream about steaks even if you have been a long-term vegetarian. Bone broth is one of the most mineral-rich and supportive things you can consume for this work. Please listen to your body as best you can as it signals you. At the minimum, you will need to increase healthy fats and oils as this will highly support the brain and neurological system to handle this work, even if you are being called toward a more vegetable-based diet. Mineral-rich foods and supplementation are also recommended. You will also likely be called to clean up your diet of processed foods and refined sugar. Coconut water is beneficial to replenish after healing or channeling sessions.

Of course, the keys are your personal, energetic practices, meditation, prayer, and taking time for rest. Your physical body is a priority. This work is no good if it is taking you out. Occasionally, I have seen people undergo a healing crisis because their body rebalances quickly. Some people call this ascension sickness or awakening flu. This might include flu-like symptoms, body aches, fever, exhaustion, or other physical illness symptoms. This is because the higher work needs to move through a clearer vessel, and you must clean up your act. If you are still recreationally using any form of stimulants, drugs, or alcohol, you might get a wake-up call to change things quickly. Increased heat during these works can stress the kidneys, so you might need more kidney and adrenal support, as the adrenals are directly connected to the kidneys. There are supportive vitamin and herbal formulas, often containing ashwagandha, holy basil, and B vitamins. You can also seek advice from a naturopath or Chinese Medical Doctor specializing in herbs.

Traditional Western esotericists believed that this type of work must only be done by those who exhibited strength and toughness to endure the exceptional forces required to transmit. Serious training was always done in the esoteric mystery schools to build physical endurance and tenacity. You might not think physical exercise would be a key to mediumship work, but it is. Running, hiking, pushups, squats, weight training, and martial arts are highly supportive. They also believed this work should only be done by those with a solid connection to life. This means a strong thread is connecting the soul to the body. Those who are highly depressive, weak, and not connected to their physical body should take great care. They are vulnerable to being taken over by entities or overwhelmed by energetic forces.

So, while you might think that what is required for this type of work is a very spiritual, ethereal nature, it is recommended that you become as solid, rooted, and grounded as possible. This means that you can tune into your physical and energetic bodies and root, track, and move your own energy successfully. You must know yourself fully so that you are aware of what isn't you.

As I said, "Today might not be a good day to be a shaman," so too, today might not be a good day to do any channeling work. If you are exhausted, ill, or unstable, give yourself a break, rest, and return later.

8

WORKING THE
PSYCHIC CENTERS

The light was always there. I just couldn't see it yet.

You have built energy in the belly (Lower Dantian) to support this work. Then, you opened your heart (Middle Dantian) to receive energy and master discernment. The Upper Dantian in the head is responsible for your intuitive and psychic perceptions, but it must be balanced with the other energy centers to bring through true visions. Awareness of and meditation on the upper center will help open your channel, but you need to be firm in the lower centers to avoid destabilizing your system. Work with the following areas slowly and give yourself time to notice your experiences. Always source your energy into the lower centers before going to the upper points. Practice returning your energy to your belly in between and do supportive, grounding practices to support stabilization. Don't discount the potency of these simple practices.

Start these meditations by bringing conscious presence to each area and feeling as though you are breathing through or gently looking through that area. Remember to massage, tap, and energetically cleanse these areas regularly.

Third Eye

The area between your brows and slightly above them, "Heaven's Eye," allows you to observe the subtle spiritual realms and spiritual light to illuminate the inner chambers of the upper center. This is the front gate of the sixth chakra.

Crown

Here is the upper gate of the central channel and the seventh crown chakra. From here, you can connect to Source energy and receive messages from the Divine.

Back of the Skull

Below the occipital protuberance at the base of the skull is the antenna where you receive messages, "God's Mouth." This is where information comes in, and you receive spirits in trance-channeling states. This is the back gate of the sixth chakra. This area is one of the most helpful to work with for channels. Massage this area, feeling underneath the skull while looking up and down. Again, clean this regularly through tapping and swiping.

Center of the Brain, Pineal Gland

This tiny gland located in front of the cerebellum is the gland of telepathic communication. It reads projected thoughts. It shrinks as we age and is affected and calcified by chemicals and lack of use. Its awakening is supported by vibrating the bones of the skull in toning and singing practices that focus sound into the head.

Chimney

This area is located above and behind the back of the skull area. Imagine it like the chimney of your fireplace. You receive spiritual information from here, and energy is released to the Divine. This area must be cleaned regularly by tapping, using your hands to clear upward, and visualizing any stuck or dark energy flowing up to the light while breathing and focusing on the exhaled breath. Be sure to cleanse from the top of the shoulders, the neck and back of the head, and the entire area behind. These regular clearings make a huge difference in brain fog, headaches, neck pain, and exhaustion.

[Practice 45: Clearing and Opening the Upper Center]

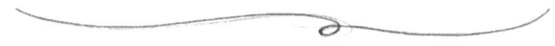

9

CONFUSING ASPECTS OF WORKING WITH GUIDES AND SPIRITS

Wait? Is that a demon?

Working with guides and other beings isn't straightforward, as they may not show up in the ways you expect. You may have watched films or heard others share their encounters and assume it will be similar for you. Additionally, you may believe you will receive information in the way you imagine they receive it. When someone says, "I see" or "I hear," you may think they have a very concrete sensory experience. They might use those words but have a different relationship to what that means in this context. We often receive guidance through feeling states, subtle knowings, and impressions that are like images but have much less substance than we think they should.

Many assume that opening their channel and meeting their guides will give them answers to all life's questions, and they will be able to ask precisely what to do in every situation and have a hotline for consistent clarity. While you will develop clarity and receive important guidance, these beings don't give you all the answers. They want you to learn to use your intuition and inner guidance. They are slowly getting to know you—feeling into your intentions, being aware of gifts and wounds—which might cause you to give up your spiritual pursuits or fall victim to ego-driven decision-making. They realize that a long-term mentorship strategy will serve you best, even if this sometimes means seeming to abandon you as you develop your capacities and heal.

Negative Experiences with Spirit Entities

Demons can be our greatest teachers. I say this because most people I have seen deal with the darker forces have become stronger and more capable. One of my teachers says that our higher guides oversee our touches with the demonic as we learn about spirits and ourselves and receive instruction in boundaries and sovereignty. These experiences are often training grounds and initiations for powerful practitioners. After all, it is hard to confront issues in others without personal knowledge. This isn't to say that you necessarily want or need these experiences or that they will be a part of your path.

When working with great quantities of light, you'll naturally attract a grand array of beings. Some are curious. They want to know what is going on. Some are simply past or future projections; some might even be embodied humans currently spirit traveling, and some might be Elementals, Nature Spirits, or ghosts. Many help and guide, and these are the ones that you'll mainly focus on in your work. Many are passing through like tourists in the realms. Others are there to harm in some way actively.

The more you tap into your spiritual and energetic awareness and perception, the more you will be aware of other beings. You don't need to know everything about them. You don't need to engage with all of them. Often, they are on their path and will come and go quickly and quietly. When you are in the treatment space and intend to be an open channel and heighten your awareness, or in medicine space or deep meditation, you might be aware of them in a way you have not been before.

Disembodied beings are everywhere, all the time. Your senses block them out to avoid being overwhelmed and confused. When the subtle abilities are opening, you may experience uncomfortable heightened sensations or an abundance of beings. It will become manageable as you gain proficiency in your energetic boundaries, sovereignty, and clarity on how you engage with your psychic awareness.

Some individuals with heightened sensitivity see dark entities around others in public places such as buses or on the street. They have asked whether it is their responsibility to aid in removing these entities from the affected individual, as they may be causing distress.

Consent in healing work is necessary. You might feel obligated to help others who appear to be suffering, but they haven't contracted you to do so. In this, you could pull dark energies off people all day long. They might feel better for a bit, but their thoughts, actions, and energetic patterns are such that another being, much like the last, will come to them shortly. It is important in this work to tune into your guides and see if working with someone is the appropriate course of action. You can put yourself in danger if you seek to shift something for someone that is a part of their karmic experience. This means that if someone is not doing the inner work to address what is attracting the dark energies, they create the karmic address for the energy to remain.

I had a client who worked in a clinical psychiatric setting for people experiencing mental health crises. Spirits, beings, and energy were not part of the program. She would notice how people would seem to be taken over, and on occasion, she would clear the being or call in angelic presence, and the person would become lucid again. Yet soon, the person would be back where they were before. Sometimes, they were seemingly worse. Because there wasn't a holistic treatment protocol, engaging the consent of the patient and incorporating belief systems that resonate with the afflicted, spiritual, shamanic, and energetic work had less chance of lasting effect.

We have lost our connections to the shamanic ways. They are not considered socially acceptable treatments in most standard mental health and addiction recovery programs. Shifts are occurring where ceremonial, plant medicine, and traditional healing modalities are being implemented with success in more areas. But, it isn't an easy task to introduce and do these therapies with the mentally ill. They may suffer from spirit attachments but also have many other issues and are vulnerable to attack because of the stored trauma in their systems and their lifestyles. Spiritual and energetic clearings can be very supportive, but returning to an abusive home of rage and addictions will be like dropping them back into a toxic soup. The sensitive one in the family often expresses the underlying darkness around the family and community. The work that we do is holistic. It must encompass not only the spiritual or the energetic but also the thoughts and actions of the individual seeking support. Unfortunately, many don't have the resources or support systems to help them with this often long road of recovery and change.

I don't want to discourage you from addressing attachments in those with mental health issues. But, as I said, it must be a holistic journey that encourages shifts in all areas of life and often requires support from other practitioners.

Who Are These Beings Anyway?

I want to briefly overview entities you may encounter while exploring the spiritual realms. Being aware of them is essential to aiding in your growth and identifying them when a client encounters them.

Guides and Teachers

These are the angels and other guides, including animal spirits, galactic beings, and the ascended masters who have dedicated their spiritual evolution after death toward supporting humanity. They are here to do exactly what you would expect. They can access higher realms of wisdom and guide, teach, and assist. They might be familiar culturally, but they are often unique to you in how they present. You have many guides and teachers. They operate under free will and support you when you ask for it. They often speak in the subtle messages of synchronicity.

Mediumship Mentors

This non-physical being assists and mentors you to understand and efficiently, safely, and effectively be used as a channel and medium for healing and illumination. This guide focuses on helping you bring through spiritual information to help others. This mentor is much the same as you would describe a physical mentor here on Earth. They work closely with you to help you develop and advance your spiritual and energetic gifts and awareness. This mentor assists channeling and mediumship works by acting as an intermediary for the beings you bring through. This makes it easier for your body to assimilate the process of channeling. They act as a bridge between you and other beings, supporting your sense of safety and ease with new frequencies. The mediumship mentor works with you closely, teaching you over time. They are invited in through devotion, intention, and request. They feel your authenticity and heart and offer their wisdom and guidance.

You decided to take up the job of coming to Earth to be in a body, forgetting everything that happens between lifetimes. Your mentor is a trusted friend and partner in these works stationed on the other side to help guide you, illuminate your gifts, and shepherd you into alignment so that you can do the work of bringing more light and love to this planet. This is accomplished by channeling through the higher realms of consciousness, giving people access to love, connection, and awareness of Spirit. These guides help you understand the spiritual realms and your own emerging gifts. They keep you safe in the confusing world of the unseen.

If you want to meet and work with your mediumship mentor, make this an intention while meditating. Converse with this being and ask for guidance. You have free will and must ask for help and then sit and be present with what comes through, even if slowly. You might say: "I request the support of a mediumship mentor. I wish to be of service to the Light and an open channel to Divine Love. I wish to understand my mediumship and develop."

Healers, Shamans, or Doctor Spirits

If you are a healer, you'll have healing spirits to call upon in your work. These beings are former physicians, nurses, alchemists, shamans, medicine people, and healers. They often have been embodied, so they are easy to work with and integrate. They may also be off-planet beings with healing knowledge and experience.

Some people have trouble considering that they will work with a 'doctor' spirit because they have a negative view of doctors and Western medicine. If you notice this comes up for you when you hear the term doctor spirit, consider that these guides hold a positive intent toward healing and wellness on every level. They might be associated with a lineage you are familiar with or from another one entirely.

My personal healing guides are mostly shamanic in nature. When I do hands-on healing work, they are with me throughout the session and have taught me about singing and sound, extracting through my hands and mouth, how not to allow toxic energy to enter me in that process, and different techniques I have not learned elsewhere. I had to accept the weird things I was guided to do in sessions, especially the dramatic coughing and energetic vomiting that would occur when working, seeing and feeling foreign objects in the body, and the strange sounds, movements, and songs. I have been surprised to learn that the techniques I have been guided to do are common in other traditions. It has been validating to me to read about or see traditional healers utilize similar strategies. Hearing them discuss why they work this way or where they learned this, they always acknowledge the spirits that inform their work.

Your healing guides may be ancient Chinese practitioners informing you of meridian lines to work with or Chinese herbs to employ. They might be midwives and European folk healers instructing you on their herbal lineage or ways that were lost through so much Western medical thought. Perhaps they are African healers speaking to you of their traditional ways. You have the opportunity to expand as a healer by listening deeply, noticing the guidance that arises, and asking for more information and support. You can even get quite specific in your requests to work with particular types of healing guides based on the work you are currently called to do.

You work with them because:

- They can do more dangerous work. You don't have to do all the heavy lifting in your practice.

- When working with them in session, you are safer and more protected. You are less likely to take on others' energy; they assist in moving the energy out of this plane.

- They guide and give more information; they might even have helpful medical or herbal suggestions. Many experience them as guiding their hands or speaking to them while they work.

- They teach techniques of their lineage and how to work with plant and animal spirits for healing.

- They help perform psychic surgery and extractions.

[Practice 46: How to Begin Working with a Doctor Spirit]

The Others

In an open channel state, you connect to beings and energies through your nervous system. If it doesn't feel good or in alignment, stop. Don't lower your vibration in an attempt to merge and connect more. If you feel you are coming in contact with harmful beings, do your energy practices, and don't go far from your body. Spirits can lie and trick you. Your embodiment practices, hosting a radiant inner core of light, having a strong field, and being able to listen to your gut and heart will support you in navigating these relationships. Feel free to ask spirits questions to learn more about them, and always be willing to shut down a connection that doesn't feel right. Commitment to your ethical compass and alignment with your values and purpose will help you remain connected to your essence and the beings that resonate. Do not be deluded by the trappings of power, fame, desire, greed, lust, envy, or control. Spirits can sniff out your weaknesses and use them against you.

As I have said, awareness of risks in this work does not mean focusing on what might go wrong. For the most part, you will have beneficial experiences. Don't drag yourself down by being overly fearful or obsessive about difficult experiences.

Not all experiences ascribed to spirits are that. Your psyche also speaks to you and creates internal images or even, at times, external images that might be misinterpreted. If you are struggling with mental health issues, you may project your inner critic or pain in a way that feels external. I am offering you ways to work with your consciousness and build your field of light and internal reserves, whether you have a spiritual or a mental issue.

Mocking Spirits

These lower-level beings aren't at the level of complex consciousness as vicious spirits or demons. (see below) They are opportunists who don't have a larger picture plan of attack. They feed by getting you to release negative emotions and thought forms by "mocking" you. They don't have a lot of new lines, so they use the same ones over and over, "You're a loser," "No one loves you," "You're ugly," "You're stupid." You think these are your own as they play on repeat. This lowers your vibration and pulls you away from your purpose.

Taking a moment to consider a thought might not be yours can be enough to release it. This pause allows you to be present and do something different instead of repeating an old pattern. The old pattern would be to repeat the thought, react emotionally, and stir up negative feelings about yourself. This might culminate in deciding not to move forward on a project or advocate for your well-being. You set yourself free by instigating a pause when you come across this pattern. You no longer live reactively but choose what you allow to plant in your consciousness. With repetition, you break a cycle that brings you down.

It doesn't matter if it is your thoughts or an influencing factor if you work with your consciousness to shift your response. If this is your psyche and not a spirit, the self-degrading thought was encoded from someone else, such as a parent, peer, or partner. With that awareness, you see that these beliefs aren't yours. They are not a part of your intrinsic nature. An external force has installed them. It is crucial to release beliefs that align with these negative statements while building confidence and self-esteem through self-care practices and expressing your truth, boundaries, and creative energy.

Destructive, Vicious Spirits and Demons

These beings are more evolved dark entities. They feed off pain, fear, regret, resentment, rage, and desire. They can latch onto a family for generations, and some were called into service by dark sorcerers or witches long ago. Many cultures have collective beliefs in these demons; some even work with and feed them. They can be used to hurt others if you can bring them under your control, but in the end, this will always come back to harm you.

These beings love addictions and abusive homes. They hang around in places steeped in violence, bars, drug dens, and gambling halls. There are places you will not want to be when you are psychically open because you pick up on these beings and the residual energy of actions, thoughts, and emotions in the space, which doesn't feel good. They prefer someone who is resonant with them or is weakened, so even if you find yourself in a less-than-ideal situation, do not let fear take over. Some of these beings can be removed and sent into a portal of light or worked with to move on from a place or person, but it isn't recommended to interact with these entities without proper training.

People often give more power to these entities by constantly fearing them or conflating that every spiritual or energetic experience or moment of bad fortune is because of them. You may experience something that frightens you, but it could be a misinterpretation of a strong energy. If your nervous system is used to being overwhelmed and dysregulated, you might interpret beneficial energies as a danger.

Your work in this book: grounding, sourcing, cleansing, and purification, and becoming a grateful, radiant blessing to the world will change your life circumstances, karmic address (what you do and create that is a vibrational match for a negative entity), and influences from these beings. Your focus on maintaining a strong center and sovereign state will help ward them off. Movement, sound, and breath practices heal your nervous system, so you have a larger zone of resiliency to operate in as you come in contact with different energies. Stating your boundaries, saying no, and making it absolutely clear they are not allowed in your space is vital. Call upon light, the angelic forces, and the highest spiritual beings to help clear the space. Be certain in your power and protection.

Wrathful Deities

These are often mistaken for vicious entities because they are seen or experienced as scary and dark, but they shock you into growth. They are fierce and forceful and hope to remove obstacles in your life. You may miss a needed message or transmission from these beings because you see things from a surface level. Move through your fears and wounds and sit with any encounters from a calm and present place without jumping to conclusions. They can represent the direct and powerful force you need to move through blocks to your spiritual evolution and growth. Be curious in your interactions to determine what you are experiencing and what you can learn. Religious programming can impede the ability to consider that something that appears fierce or challenging might be beneficial, signaling inner work to be done. These beings might startle you, but they are not likely to override your free will, manipulate you, or seek to incorporate through you without permission.

This is another reason to focus on your work to remain grounded and sourced with light and energy. As you cultivate a presence of safety that arises from and through you, you can be with challenging moments of introduction with a powerful being. You may even witness your intimidation transforming into awe and wonder.

Elementals and Nature Spirits

These old and powerful beings are associated with the elements or places in nature. They can be disturbed by destroying or disrespecting natural areas. They are guardians, which is one reason we walk lightly and respectfully in nature and make offerings when in their domain. They can be allies and powerful healing spirits that show up during ceremonies in their realms.

There are spirits of the land and spirits of the home that are often helpful and enjoy human presence. It is important to acknowledge these spirits in your regular practices, placing flowers, food, water, herbs, incense, or other offerings on your altar for them. They can be very supportive beings that help your life run smoothly.

Ancestors

Ancestors from your genetic lineage can be influencing forces whether you consciously work with them or not. I encourage you to have an ancestral altar where you can place pictures of relatives who have passed (don't include pictures of any living people), flowers, loved foods and drinks, and appreciated items. Consider what your people's staple grains and foods were. Did they rely on oats, rice, corn, beer, wine, or vodka? Don't put an ancestor altar in the bedroom, as they can disrupt sleep and intimacy. Speak with them, light candles for them, and pray for them. Ask for support from beneficial ancestors. Ask them to teach you about ancient ways, herbalism, growing food, or anything else they might be interested in. You can ask them to support you in letting go of long-held family wounds and inherited trauma. You can also make prayers that your ancestors be relieved of pain, suffering, or guilt, and pray for anyone whom your ancestors have harmed, asking for forgiveness for them and blessings for their descendants. Through these prayers, offerings, and presence, you may find relief in your own life or illumination on what you have been carrying that is not really yours.

There are also ancestors of lineages. When you study a lineage, you can ask to connect to the holders of that lineage and, with deep respect and humility, ask for their instruction in your meditations, practices, and dreams.

Ghosts

These souls have departed the human body but not human experiences. There are two major classifications of ghosts: benign and malignant.

Benign ghosts are phantoms, free-floaters who are often lost, confused, delusional, or desire to guide and protect the living. They may be confused because they died unexpectedly and are unaware they have passed on, as in the case of some victims of violent deaths. They may need to be informed of their current situation. Some lack closure and seek that before leaving this plane. They may show up to give messages to loved ones, warn people, or clear their conscience. Many times, they simply need to be heard. To support them, you can request and open a portal of light and help them find and go through it. They are sometimes scared to leave their family or unsure of the light as they don't believe in such things. A conversation often helps, and you can call on beings to support such as Archangel Azrael, who helps transport souls to the other side. Archangel Michael is often called up upon in these situations to support the process and protect you. If they don't want to go to the other side, you must state they cannot remain in your space or attach to or bother you or your family.

Malignant ghosts are angry, malicious, destructive, and mischievous, responsible for hauntings, psychic attacks, and poltergeist activity. They become this way because they are obsessed or grief-stricken. Something is keeping them here, and it may be addictions, intense negative emotions such as anger or fear that they can't let go of, or an unhealthy connection to a living person or place. They are searching. They might search for a person, a body, or energetic food. Some can overshadow thoughts, obstruct or block spiritual progress, or frighten and shock. You can try the same techniques as I have listed before, but you may want to leave them alone if possible.

Hungry ghosts are a subset of 'ghosts' with huge mouths and no stomachs, so they are always hungry. They are responsible for when people always want more. They might desire more food, clothes, cars, money, whatever. They are the manifestation of greed in an energetic form. They can attach to a person who craves what they crave, making addictions worse.

There are other beings with different forms that you might recognize over time. You may see them as overlays or shadows enveloping someone's body. They may arise in your consciousness when you tune into someone. You may notice that people with specific issues seem to have similar attachments. Your experience will depend on how your psychic abilities are expressed. You may never see anything, but you might feel, know, and be able to communicate with what is there.

Thought Forms

Not all "spiritual" experiences are what they seem. This is because thoughts have energy, and what we experience as an entity could be a perception of the energetic matrix created by thoughts and feelings. Thoughts are generated in our energy centers and travel out of the front of the body and into the world. They attract similar energy, gain power, and then return to the body to feed us with the same energy we have been putting out. Therefore, it's crucial to transform your relationship with your thoughts, relaxing your identification with them. You are empowered by choosing to witness your thoughts and see them as energy passing through. As you develop the ability to take a pause and be present with what you are witnessing, you can choose to modify them, replacing lower vibrational ones with those that align with your higher self.

Thoughts hold immense power. When you focus intensely on them and fuel them with emotional energy, they are on their way to becoming a full-fledged entity. This thought form will resonate with a specific frequency, feeding off you, and when it is powerful enough, it goes out into the world to feed more. The more emotional energy it consumes, the more powerful it becomes.

Many people are weighed down by their thought forms and

those picked up from the collective. The cleansing and purification practices help clear these thought form energies while enabling you to develop new thoughts and beliefs. It's important to note that the mental wavelengths of those in your social circle and home tend to merge, forming a larger thought form matrix. This energetic thought matrix is why you may feel worse in densely populated areas due to the thought and emotional congestion you are picking up on. This collective field enhances the effects of media as you connect to an energy grid with those producing, experiencing, and watching.

A manifestation that arises from the collective thoughts of a specific group is called an egregor. These collective thought forms can be extremely strong. This is why group rituals are so powerful, and mobs can arise in generally peaceful people. Knowing this, we can create powerful, intentional, positive egregors through group prayer, meditation, singing, and ceremonies. These have positive effects on the individuals involved and the collective.

Awareness of this can assist you in asking pertinent questions of your client, tracking thoughts and feelings they express regularly, and guiding them towards overcoming old patterns and engaging in new ways of being that align with their values. They can become more conscious of their surroundings and how the individuals they associate with can impact them.

I have discussed how you can use your imagination to affect your energy, body, and health. To imagine is to create. We are extraordinary creators; our focus and attention determine where energy flows. We have worked to stabilize ourselves so we aren't lost in imaginings and "ghost syndrome."

The Subconscious and Ghost Syndrome

The subconscious mind can bring up energetic visions and projections, parts of the self brought to the conscious mind to be dealt with. These visions can take many forms and are often linked to intense, suppressed emotions. Many experience this when encountering "demons" in meditation, dreams, or medicine work. These projections diminish as one works through suppressed emotions, releasing them from the body and energy field.

As previously discussed, energetic deviations can cause hallucinations and illusions. This is why you are guided to focus on the lower energy centers, releasing trauma and emotions from the body and stabilizing your energy. Without proper self-work and cultivating energy in the lower centers, diving too deeply into psychic and spiritual practices may lead to mistaking these experiences for encounters with entities. This is often observed in individuals who have not yet engaged in stabilizing healing work and are doing a lot of medicine work or focusing on opening the third eye. It is possible to do too much energy and spiritual development work if you jump in suddenly, doing several hours a day of advanced practices with no previous experience, especially without a guide.

The power of the subconscious mind is immense. It's crucial to focus on raising your vibration through positive thoughts and deeds as you release judgments and attachments. This will ensure your desires and fears don't create false perceptions or inner voices that lead you astray.

10

DISCERNMENT

Discernment is a function of the entire body.

C an you distinguish between positive and negative forces when receiving messages or inspiration? Are you clear when messages are helpful as opposed to dangerous? Can you follow your intuitive guidance as you move through the world?

The ability to have effective discernment in every area of life asks you to be grounded, sourced, clear, and embodied. This is also supported by cleansing and performing vibration-raising practices in the purification processes. Movement, breath, and sound reintroduce you to your embodied presence as you heal old trauma and nervous system dysregulation. Without this foundation, you might be unable to "hear" what your body is telling you. If you haven't cleared old emotional baggage from your heart, you won't be able to be fully present to its wisdom shining through.

The mind can make up all sorts of fantasies and delusions. The gut, the collective intuition of your lower centers and organs, and your heart have clearer wisdom. Become an expert at tuning into your body, asking questions, listening, and receiving answers. Act on those answers and see the results. Allow your physical and energetic practices to relieve you of old stagnations in the body. Free yourself from reactive dysregulation and chaos. Find your centered presence and practice maintaining it. This is the time to explore the spirit realms. Work in the unseen worlds can get messy if you are ungrounded, disembodied, and operating from harmful old programs, traumas, and patterns.

This is also why choosing your guides and practitioners wisely is crucial, as many people—even medicine ceremony facilitators—

have little grasp or concept of the spiritual or energetic realms, and ceremonies, retreats, and energy practices can open you up quickly. If you keep mastering the basics, you will have greater stability for a more significant opening that will support your path and healing process. Otherwise, you might have to backtrack for the more foundational work, which is challenging when your energy body is running "too hot," or your spiritual experiences have become overwhelming.

You might go your whole life without interacting with the unseen realms, but the question here is, what the heck do you do if you come in contact with beings in your work?

If something does show up, checking in and practicing discernment is essential. Ask questions.

- Is this congruent with a feeling of love and light?

- Does this serve your highest and best?

- Is this useful?

- Does this limit or control?

- Does this feel expansive or contractive?

- Is this offering "all the answers" or encouraging your evolution and development?

Feel the emotions and energy that are present in the interaction.

  » Do they feel good?

  » Is there anger or fear under the surface?

  » Does the "mood" shift and change quickly, or does it feel

consistent, nurturing, and kind?

Feel with your heart.

> » Can this being or energy truly touch your heart, or are they touching your mind and ego?

> » Are they telling you to do things?

> » Are they rude, bossy, promising you things, or building up your ego?

Alignment

As you do your inner work and transform your consciousness, build your energy body, and shift your vibration through your actions, words, and deeds, you will become more aligned with higher beings. These beings will be congruent with love, compassion, and grace.

You may come in contact with beings that are not in alignment with these higher aspects of being. They want to knock you off your path, drain your energy, confuse you, and keep you in your ego and mind and disconnected from your internal guidance. There is no need to live in fear, but all need discernment in these astral waters. As you become more precise and in control of your system, you will tune into different frequencies more easily. You don't prefer every radio station; the same will be true of beings and energies, and as you up-level yourself, you will naturally be tuned to higher-frequency beings.

A true being of the light will never shame you, command you, require of you, or tell you that you are the second coming of Christ. I assume you aren't. They will not offer you gold and riches. In possessions I have seen, several have come from the unconscious overuse of medicines while not focusing on inner work but on status, power, and sensational experiences and not having experienced guides. A contract is created when a being offers power, financial ease, or "spirit sex" with the person. They appeal to base desires. Over time, the being becomes more demanding and won't leave, creating havoc and eventually showing its true colors. A being of the light will never encourage hatred, abuse, addiction, or hurting yourself or others. They don't demand or impose but are ambassadors of free will and align with universal laws, even when sharing harsh truths with you.

If you come in contact with one of these beings, it is an opportunity for you to embrace the teaching moment and explore what your base desires are that have been exploited. You have received this in order to develop and heal yourself. This, along with clarity on your boundaries, intentions, and declaration of your sovereignty, is usually enough to shift the connection. Come back to your practices of cleansing, purification, grounding, and holding a strong inner core of light as an embodied, radiant being. Call upon your guides and protective beings. Remember who you are and what you stand for.

Some people are designed to attract beings that seem of a lower-level status as their systems are adept at helping these disembodied beings shift over to the light. They might be a bit lost on the way after death. They can seem sad, despondent, or scary to those with psychic gifts. This is another reason people shut down the gift of psychic sight early. While you have every right to set boundaries in these interactions, such as, "I don't want to be visited at night," it is worth inquiring about your gifts and how they are used. Part of your service may be to communicate with and help these lost souls. When you are open, you might be visited by the departed to bring messages to those still living. Mostly, these beings mean no harm. They are seeking help and realize you can interact with and support them. Setting parameters on these interactions and releasing fear of them can open up your work to a rewarding service. I highly encourage you to keep precise 'office hours' for this type of work so you are not visited and disturbed by these beings in a way that disrupts your life. Simple statements of boundaries and containers benefit most people challenged by these visitations.

Let's talk about fear and its effects. Lower-level beings are drawn to fear and feed off it. You can be aware that they exist and not live in fear. The less fear you hold in your system and the more you fully embody and trust yourself, the less effect they have on you. Fear pulls you out of your body, depletes your energy, and creates holes in your auric field. It makes you vulnerable. Obsessive rumination doesn't serve you but feeds what you seek to be free of. Focus on practices that help you feel empowered and connected to your inner light. Trust yourself and your sovereignty to shield you from negative influences.

You might also come into contact with lower-level beings to build discernment. It is part of your training, supported by your higher guides, so you can do your work with a heightened awareness of who you are working with at all times.

If in any way you feel "off" about something you come in contact with, say, "No." If a being doesn't make you feel good in your body and touches your heart, it is probably not worth connecting with anyway. This doesn't mean you might not feel extra energy, goosebumps, or temperature changes when interacting with beings; those might feel uncomfortable in their newness. Those naturally inclined toward incorporated mediumship (when a spirit enters the body) can have even more intense physical sensations. These might include heart pain, nausea, or as if the inside of your body is being stretched beyond its previous capacity. Again, remember you are in control, and slow down or stop the process if you feel overwhelmed.

You might also experience a nervous system response to heightened sensations. This means past experiences are triggering you, and you might dissociate or shut down to manage the sensations. This is when you know you need to focus on your practices. Movement, breath, and sound will support you in increasing your zone of resiliency. This builds your ability to be uncomfortable and experience heightened sensations. If you feel that coming in contact with spiritual forces is triggering you, address it immediately by inhaling quickly through the nose and then letting the breath out long and slow to reactivate your parasympathetic nervous system.

Build your team of guides slowly and with reverence. With time, you will be able to track how certain feeling sensations are associated with specific beings. This helps you trust your guides and yourself. As I have said, there is no need to invoke every deity known to man as this may cause more confusion and overwhelm. Practice intentionally closing your channel, stating your boundaries, and maintaining your center by calming your nervous system through simple breathwork and developing your inner core of light.

11

SAFETY AND PROTECTION

I am Your Love that protects me here.

P eople take precautions during certain activities in the gross or "real" world. Doctors wear gloves, individuals who prepare food for others wash their hands and utilize specialized tools, and those involved in art or construction often wear respiratory masks and helmets. You can do all these jobs without taking these now standard industry precautions. You can succeed in your endeavors, but issues will arise at a certain point. In the past, successful surgeries were performed without knowledge of germs, but some resulted in severe infections and sepsis. Similarly, many talented artists who were exposed to toxic compounds later developed cancer or experienced mental health issues.

It is the same in the subtle realms. Without basic preventive procedures, we can leave ourselves and the people we work with open to infection, disease, irritation, feeling overwhelmed, or more serious issues that might not immediately be noticed. They are compounded over time. Like attracts like, and a buildup eventually overwhelms the system and reserves.

Some mistakes are when we believe:

- All is light.

- I can't be infiltrated.

- I can work anytime, anywhere.

- I don't have to maintain a personal practice.

- I don't have to cleanse and purify.

If you acknowledge light, you must also acknowledge dark. There is balance in all things. You contain both shadow and light. It doesn't mean you are bad or wrong because this is true, and learning to be with these energies illuminates your inner work. When used correctly, both are signals and invitations for learning and growth. Once again, I encourage you to come from a place of empowered light, love, and joy. There is no need to fear anything that arises. It is most often there to teach you about yourself.

When you focus on reaching through to the highest realms in meditation, you are safer than when working in the different planes that hold the information, ancestors, energies, lost soul parts, past life codes, and beings you tune into during healing. This is why you are learning the practices that support working in these more confusing realms.

So, what are some of the tools you need to remain calm, centered, and present even in the face of disturbing or overwhelming experiences? Many have already been discussed. Here is a checklist to remember when working in these realms:

Body and Field: Practices from previous sections: centering, grounding, sourcing, cleansing and purification, boundaries, and awareness.

Space: Practices from Cleansing and Purification and Sacred Container: smudges and resins, sound, energy work.

Consciousness: Focusing your attention, raising your vibration, and shifting your thoughts. "I am not my thoughts and feelings."

Prayer: "I ask for assistance." "I pray for . . ."

Invocations: "I call upon and invoke the presence of my healing guides and angels."

Declarations: "I am a sovereign being. I don't give permission to lower-level beings or harmful spirits to be a part of my reality in any way. I don't accept any energy of a lower vibration."

Nothing of a lower vibration can enter something (or someone) of a higher vibration. This is why you work to raise your vibration. It isn't the right time to channel when you are sick or tired. Keep your food and water pure, and live your life with integrity. The more you clean yourself, the higher level of beings will come through. Deception, raging at others, and other negative shadow behaviors must be addressed. If you haven't cleared old emotional and energetic blockages, beings will be attracted to the garbage in your system and not be of the highest vibration. Lower-level beings may seem confusing or "off," imparting information but nothing helpful. There is little reason to bring through information that isn't helpful to your life.

While you are committed to inner work, you don't have to be perfect. There is no need to force happiness. Don't shame yourself if you still have pain, illness, issues, or struggles. A focused presence with all aspects of yourself and devotion to embodied awareness will support your ability to experience and process any and all emotions. Anger channeled effectively gives you access to understanding your boundaries and can be a creative force that compels you to change. Anger can motivate you to stand up for justice and take right action. Grief teaches about love and the power of feeling deeply and caring for others and the world. Suppressing emotions is dangerous as they remain inside your body and aren't used to fuel your life. Use the tools in this book to support energetically clearing the emotions that keep you stuck while engaging with your consciousness to discover who you want to be and act from that place. Again, this is not about repressing your emotions or enforcing toxic positivity on yourself or others.

If you feel you have picked something up (an energetic, emotional, or spirit attachment), return to the earlier work: shaking, cleansing, grounding, sourcing, and purifying. Create a portal and release anything that isn't you. Use the practices that work for you; return to gratitude and prayer. Change yourself, your thoughts, and your way of being so there is no resonant energy with the intrusive force. Make the light so bright that there is no reason for them to stay.

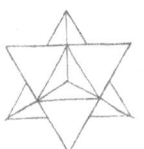

RELEASING

I release that which does not serve my highest and best from my body.

I release that which does not serve my highest
and best from my auric field.

I am the only one allowed inside of this body.

12

YOU ARE A UNIQUE CHANNEL

Every person receives, processes, and translates differently.

Every system is designed uniquely. As many puzzle pieces are shaped differentially and come together to create a larger picture, so too do your unique gifts together create a larger mission of healing and awakening. Often, you will wish to have a different gift or path.

Some will channel words or writings, or beings will come through in large movements. For others, profound information will emerge with little change to their physical form, voice, or other aspects of being. For some, opening their terminal will be a radical, intense, sweat-inducing event that will shake them to the core. For some, their channel will be expressed through creations, business, or even sex and relationships. Some have visions, hear, or feel information, while others simply know.

Sometimes, when you receive guidance, it may seem like your own internal voice. Consider that your guides are trying to reach you in a way that will be easily assimilated into your being. As a child, you may have shut down voices that didn't sound like your own, fearing them and what they meant by being there. So, your guides will speak to you through your own internal voice. Of course, it isn't always the case that the internal voice is a guide. Negative thoughts and voices would never come from an enlightened master or guide. Sometimes, these voices could come from lower-level energetic beings, and your job is to learn to discern between the two or many, as the case may be. When a voice comes into your head, ask if it can touch your heart. Is it true to your heart and the highest expressions of light and love? This will help you discern whether this voice is one that you should listen to or one that you should flick off of your energetic system and be rid of. This takes time to master.

Don't compare yourself to others when it comes to receiving information or providing healing. It is wise to study and learn from others, but it's crucial to recognize and master your unique system. Don't train yourself out of your authentic expression. Embrace your true, natural self to make progress in your explorations. Don't worry about how you appear or sound to yourself or others. This may be challenging if you struggle with being seen and heard by others. Being witnessed as a channel is a vulnerable experience. When you open your channel, it may seem strange or weird. Understand that these feelings are self-imposed judgments. Don't worry if your expression is different from others. Each puzzle piece has its unique frequency that contributes to the bigger picture. Some express energetically, indicating your role in processing energy and bringing in upgrades to the energetic systems of those on earth. This may manifest in various ways, from dramatic to imperceptible.

Once you've fully accepted yourself, the being that you are, the way you work, how your channel performs, and your healing gifts are allowed to be expressed; you will be on the road to mastery. Come from a space of full acceptance, relax, and allow what is supposed to move through you. If you are constantly comparing yourself and trying to make your channel perform a particular way, you will do a disservice to yourself, your path, and those waiting for you. As a plant expresses itself uniquely through its blooms, fruit, size, and structure, you are uniquely designed to offer your gifts to the world. Learn from others, grow, and take in information, but don't let it distract you from your most authentic expression. Take in only as much as you need, and allow your guides and carefully chosen mentors to bring you into alignment. If you don't feel resonance with your teacher, look elsewhere. Not all teachings are for all people. In the end, you are the teacher, you are the guidance, and you are the creation. If you believe in all three, you will create magic.

13

PRECISION AND SURRENDER

Powerful work is emergent, dynamic, and yet consistent.

C hanneling and healing work is a delicate balance and dance between precision and surrender. Some are more controlled and process-oriented, so surrender is the edge to lean into. Others are more open and flowing and easily slip into altered states of consciousness. If this is you, your practice is to develop precision in your work and practices. This means finding clarity, developing the ability to drop in and out of altered states more proficiently, and cultivating heightened awareness to help others integrate your work.

Surrender allows authentic expression as you tap into your ability to bring through what you are designed to. Despite this, surrender can be daunting for some, who may fear the possibility of danger or being overwhelmed. These concerns often stem from a deeper fear of death and complete annihilation. They can also be patterns of control instilled from a lifetime of living in chaotic situations. When these feelings arise, it is important to remember you are divinely held and protected, repeat that to yourself regularly, and breathe out anything in your body that does not currently feel in alignment with that statement.

When precision and surrender play together, you have a dynamic, effective way of working with people. You have consistency and can rely on your work unfolding as it should.

When I began expressing my authentic self, I was constantly concerned my work wouldn't "turn on" and I would have nothing to offer. I imagined myself standing there frozen. I didn't have the tools and strategies to understand the consistent ways that my system functioned so I could be effective and precise. Frankly, I was all over the place. This is why I spent years unwinding this process and offer it here.

What Builds Precision?

- Daily practices

- Working on yourself

- Working with other people

- Understanding the techniques and triggers that drop you into a pure state of presence and healing or a trance state.

- Practicing consciously opening and closing your channel.

- Understanding the energetics of your work and how to focus your energy

- Intention

What Builds Surrender?

- Trauma healing and nervous system repair

- Building energy in the Lower Dantian

- Doing work around trust and feeling safe

- The Archetype work outlined in Chapter 1

- Working with Earth energy

- Regular experiences outside your comfort zone

- Dance and ecstatic and trance-inducing states

- Intention

14

REGULATING THE CHANNEL

Mastery means knowing what you need and when you need it.

There is great responsibility in being a channel. Owning the honor requires development and mastery. This means studying yourself and the triggers, boundaries, and processes that make it possible, comfortable, consistent, and functional for your life. This is not something that is happening to you but something you choose to interact with from an empowered place.

Down-regulation: If Your Channel Is Too Open

When you open the channel through intentional practices, meditations, substances, or a spontaneous awakening or re-opening from childhood, the system can be overwhelmed by too much information.

As an open channel, you are a beacon of light to the spiritual realms. Imagine a high-power antenna opening to every radio station on the planet—the noise would be cacophonous. You might catch a few things here and there, but it wouldn't be precise or clear. This is what many experience as they open their channels. Information comes in, but it is unclear and unreliable. Being engulfed by energy and spirits causes many to shut down to protect themselves or fight to remain open while everything feels like too much. The result is insufficient sleep, brain fog, partial messages, and a lack of trust in self and the acquired information.

When my channel opened, I was consumed by lengthy, energetically intense experiences and beings flying in any time. I didn't think I had the right or ability to control these experiences. Confronted with beings of massive size and strange vibration, which have powerful information and experiences to share, one can feel small, powerless, and at the whim and mercy of these beings. When a being came through while I was driving on the freeway, I decided to take my studies seriously and sought outside support. I searched for the right tools for me. First, I said no. I stopped channeling altogether until I understood my energy system and was in control of it. I worked on grounding and clearing my auric field and body. I began being very intentional. I started the journey I am taking you on by studying, practicing, receiving, and piecing it together as I went.

You have a right and, frankly, a duty to say no when something comes in at a time or in a way you don't want. You don't have to be open for business all the time.

All kinds of spiritual beings will be attracted to an open channel. Just because a being is on another plane or is an extra-terrestrial doesn't mean they are full of wisdom, honest, or for your best. Sometimes, they want to pop in and feel what it is like to be inside a human form because it's interesting.

These beings may not be aware of your daily needs. They feel you as an open channel point and want to come through. They may not consider you are occupied with eating, sleeping, driving, or other activities in which a channel state isn't most conducive to getting things done on the material plane. When you have declared a life of service and healing, supportive beings show up to do the work. This is beneficial, but it must also be in alignment and support of your "real" life. When you are clear, they know when they are allowed because you have invited and permitted them. This invitation process helps to ensure you are working with higher-level/frequency beings because you are setting boundaries and require consent to be in a container together. This is you declaring your free-will relationships with these beings.

This is why working on your sense of individuated sovereign identity as a channel is essential. Here is where the sovereignty work you have been doing gets real.

I am a sovereign being.

I am a sovereign being.

I am a sovereign being.

Remember This?

Repeat this regularly, tapping the solar plexus to pack in energy while breathing and expanding this area, front, back, and sides of the body. Your sovereignty and self-control should never be in question.

Being a safe channel also requires creating a solid container for the work. Here we are back in the Sacred Container. When the beings you're working with know they have a container for coming through, and you're in control of it, they are less likely to show up at inopportune moments.

Business Hours

Establish clarity regarding your availability for channeling and healing work. These are your designated business hours, and adherence to them will create a solid container. If you're designed to do this work and fail to establish a regular container, you may experience struggles instead of ease. The individualized mediumistic work you're called to do will inform the type of visitations you receive. Those helping disembodied souls to transition to the light can be more affected by this than others, as these soul forms are more likely to show up at all hours requesting help or wanting to deliver a message.

If you feel bombarded by beings and energies at inopportune times, redeclare your sovereignty, state you're not open then, and tell them to come when you have created the container for this work.

Here are some phrases that will support you. As always, I invite you to free-write to create your own powerful declarations.

- "I am the only one allowed inside this human form right now."

- "You're prohibited from entering my body unless I give you permission. You don't have permission at this time."

- "I am a conscious channel and in control at every moment."

- "I am not receiving information at this time. Thank you. I will let you know when I am working."

- "I will be available for transmissions tomorrow between 11 a.m.–5 p.m."

Yes, you can be that straightforward and "mundane."

If you have deceased people showing up for help because you are good at opening a portal and supporting them to get through it:

- "I am not working right now. I will help you tomorrow at 9 a.m. Please go away until then."

If you're being kept up at night:

- "I am not available tonight for communication. I ask that you help me receive a restful night's sleep only."

Or you can ask for upgrades:

- "I am available for upgrades to my energetic system, but I need this to occur within restful sleep."

Again, be clear that you only seek connection with those of the light who serve the highest and best.

Another helpful phrase:

- "I ask that any information be brought through with grace and ease."

Shamanic initiations and psychic openings can be overwhelmingly intense, and as much as you ask for help, this process of awakening might seem relentless. In such cases, examining the traumas and emotional holdings that seek to be known and processed is crucial. It is vital to look at all areas of life that need radical honesty and change. The only way out is through; for some, quick and easy isn't part of the awakening process. Practicing movement meditation has the potential to reveal insights into past lives, soul contracts, and other valuable information that can guide you on your path. It's worth inquiring about the terms of your awakening contract and why it exists. Once you know your agreement, it can illuminate where the inner work lies in shifting or accepting it. You can appeal for it to happen with more grace and ease. An appeal is a formal request for an alteration to the divine plan your soul has committed to, so be sure to have a compelling reason for requesting any modifications.

One of my clients experienced an intense shamanic awakening, during which they connected with a crucial guide and past lives through deep channeled states. As a result of this connection, they received notebooks of writings about another lifetime and remarkable healing that addressed many of their questions about themselves. This transmission needed time and attention to move through and find completion.

Many of us need to process enormous amounts of personal, collective, and ancestral karma and trauma in this lifetime. The transmutation of lower-level energies is a dark and drawn-out process that cannot be avoided. Despite your desire for everything to be easier, it is crucial to recognize the depth and difficulty of this work. It isn't as simple as turning on your channel and then being that. You are called through the work of being a channel to heal individually and for the collective.

Going Out into the "Real World"

It's understandable if you feel overwhelmed by the outside world. Crowds can be incredibly challenging when you're receiving a lot of information. Although it may seem daunting, learning how to navigate the real world in a way that works for you is possible. You don't have to enjoy being in a large crowd, but there are ways to make it more manageable. You're being called to master this to be of service.

I remember attending events and feeling overwhelmed by stimuli and information. To cope, I would keep my hands concealed in pockets or arm warmers extending down to my fingers. This was because whenever I raised my hands, they would involuntarily "turn on" and seek people out. Even the slightest touch from someone would send a jolt through my body, often resulting in a brief, altered state of consciousness. I struggled for years with workshops, Yoga classes, and events because my channel was so easily opened. Under no circumstances could I hold hands with strangers. I frequently left such gatherings or stepped outside to ground myself by placing my hands and feet on the Earth and taking deep breaths. I am proof that practices and inner work can transform your relationship with your sensitivities, and, over time, you can become capable of handling any situation.

If you struggle with this, set yourself up for success by asking for help.

- "I am not working tonight. I don't wish to receive messages or do healing work. I am off duty. I am using this time to socialize and have fun. If you have a very important message, please let me know, and I will let you know if I am available to receive it."

You can also use these gifts to your advantage.

- "I am going to an event. I am using this as a networking opportunity to meet people who are supposed to work with me. Allow those needing my medicine to cross my path, and please help me find the right words to make the connection."

You can get as specific as you want.

Up-regulation—Vibrating at A Frequency That Will Serve Your Channel

Your effectiveness is not solely determined by what you do in your work. Your being and the energy you radiate play significant roles. By occupying a higher vibration, you naturally influence others through the law of resonance. Simply being in your presence can cause radical shifts. Therefore, it is crucial to prioritize your energy and focus on raising your vibration to maximize your impact.

Realizing this, you must take responsibility for your vibration. This entails diligently attending to your physical, etheric, emotional, spiritual, and mental bodies. Once again, self-care is the name of the game. Prioritize sleep, movement, play, nutrition, nature, positive actions and thoughts, forgiveness, and being conscious of what you expose yourself to daily. This helps you stabilize and enhance your vibration. Remember, being sad, angry, or having a bad day is okay. All emotions must be acknowledged, the shadow embraced and danced with, and natural grieving processes honored.

Strive for a sensation that even amid obstacles and hardships, your decisions align with a higher vibration rather than diminishing it. This often requires research and seeking experts to guide you through supplementation, nutrition, and practices. You may find that your nervous system needs support to shift from reactivity to responding to life with the freedom of choice. This helps you look at your thoughts and how you choose to work with your consciousness and state of being. A note on my fridge says, "I am radically responsible for my state of being." When I find myself in reactivity or a doom spiral, I repeat that to myself so that I can pause and choose a different way of being. As much as we think life would be better if the conditions were different, we learn mastery through consciously shifting our state of being even when things aren't going our way.

You can also ask for help from your spirit guides and teachers. Go into meditation and let yourself sit with a particular issue or the generalized need to raise your vibration. Connect and ask your guides for information on vitamins, practitioners, and practices. You might not get an answer right away. Ask that the things you need to bring you into balance and vitality be brought into your awareness. You might then find that you meet an acupuncturist at a party, a book about a way of eating falls off the shelf when you're in a bookstore, or you receive an email with an offer to study a practice that will change your life. You might want to learn how to muscle test yourself or work with a pendulum to gain more clarity when asking questions.

You're in the process of attuning yourself. This means you must constantly attune to the virtues of truthfulness, inner peace, trust, joy, compassion, integrity, and wisdom. This life is devoted to moral refinement, study, discipline, kindness, and service. Your deepest, darkest aspects, even if they are hidden from the public, are streaming out from you and will only attract similar energies. Don't claim what isn't yours, or use what you receive to build your ego and identity. Acknowledge your streams of information and guidance with gratitude and deep respect, living your life as an offering to these beautiful connections from which you have the blessing of learning. Any information you receive from your guides and teachers is also for you, so spend time with anything you receive to integrate it fully and live your best life.

The other benefit of raising your vibration is that you will then access higher levels of information. You may receive information from a new guide who couldn't communicate with you before. It is often the case that you have initial guides who support you in opening your channel, and once you reach a certain point, you graduate to another guide who will bring in more information or healing. After a certain point, your guides can bring through more advanced information and healing work. This is because you have raised your vibration to access and hold these higher levels of consciousness.

When you're asking for help to regulate your system in either direction, to receive upgrades or new awareness, always link your requests to your soul mission and purpose. For example, you might say:

> "I desire new upgrades, in an easeful way that I can handle, so that I can be of greater service to the world, bring my healing gifts to more people, and assist in the evolution of consciousness on the planet. Thank you."

You must then give space for this to occur. This means more quiet time alone and also a commitment to sharing your gifts to see how they evolve as needed by others.

15

THE UNAWARE MEDIUM, THE ACCIDENTAL CHANNEL

The greatest art is but a transmission moving
through a practiced medium.

Many artists, creatives, scientists, and great thinkers speak of an inspired flow state that brings through their creations. Composers often state that they didn't write the music; it existed before them, and all they did was play it. These states are mediumistic. They can be connected to great wisdom, creativity, and beauty. Artists, actors, and other creatives have also been driven mad by their artistic, mediumistic states. Van Gogh, through lack of nourishment (fasting), at times sucking on his toxic (mind-altering) paintbrush, went into extended trance states producing beautiful works of art. His madness wasn't denied by him or anyone who met him.

Unaware mediumistic states can connect with unstable energies and beings. Lacking control, grounding, or context or blending addiction with these natural channeling states can create emotional instability. People can be overwhelmed by their sensitivities and abilities. Look at the people in your life. Can you recognize this anywhere?

For example, my grandmother was an incredible healer and intuitive. She came from a line of healers, but that wasn't an open path for her. She could quickly quiet a crying baby with one touch and nurse sick and wild animals back to health. She was very sensitive and uncomfortable in public, sitting with her arms crossed in a posture of protection. I can see now how her unexpressed and uncontrolled abilities left her feeling too open and vulnerable, eventually cutting off most interaction with the outside world.

How We Become Open

There are various ways we open ourselves. We can suddenly open up through breath work, movement such as ecstatic dance, shamanic trance work such as drumming, plant medicine work, meditation, prayer, yoga, sex, art, receiving healing from practitioners, and near-death experiences, to name a few. We might consciously seek higher spiritual growth but then be caught off guard by unexpected outcomes of different practices.

As I have said, mediumship is a natural human ability, and some people are more inclined toward this path. If one is unaware that they are engaging in mediumship and are consciously or unconsciously calling in beings, they can be overwhelmed by energy trying to get through their system. The sensations of mediumship can be confusing and mistaken for panic, anxiety, or other health issues.

Those who have disconnected from their physical body because of past trauma can have a more porous, open system and a more challenging time inhabiting themselves. This lack of embodiment can make mediumistic experiences harder to control. This is one reason we have focused so much on embodiment.

We have also concentrated on inner awareness and self-healing, shifting patterns and ways of being. You are attuning to beings you resonate with based on your thoughts, feelings, and behaviors. Self-destructive behavior or harming others can attract lower-vibrational beings. Engaging in addictions, especially drugs and alcohol, can create connections to low-level entities. The unaware medium may become the unconscious channel for these beings. When you think about altered states of consciousness that bring through energies and beings, you might think about the earlier examples of drumming, movement, or entheogens. But, consider the potent opening effects of a spiraling rage attack or giving oneself over to the forces of alcohol or drugs.

Places can also highly affect unaware mediums. Some are toxic, built on sacred ground or remains, or where entities have already taken up residence. Other places where terrible things have occurred drip with palpable negative energy. Over time, these places can poison sensitive people. While some may have spiritual experiences, many will have feeling states, sensations, and thoughts affected by the energies surrounding them. These thoughts are assumed to be self-sourced and, over time, become part of the person's self-talk and personality. People rarely think the negative thoughts and feelings they are experiencing might not be coming from them.

A man who came to study mediumship with me because he managed apartment buildings and was having strange experiences. He noticed that inhabitants of certain units would tend to have the same troubling issues. One unit had a string of couples addicted to drugs and alcohol. The police had been called there many times, and conflict was a common occurrence. On preparing for inhabitancy, one of his work crew was overcome by negative thoughts and feelings, and immediately went home and broke his long-standing sobriety. It was incredibly out of character for this person. My client could pick up on the negativity in this apartment. Through energetic and spiritual remediation, he was able to shift these long-held pockets of influencing energies. He worked with the spirits of the land and planted intentional allies to support the inhabitants. His and others' experiences shifted significantly.

Awareness of accidental mediumship can help you with your clients. After all, many people seek healing due to heightened sensitivity. They absorb a great deal and may struggle with maintaining proper boundaries. They don't understand that their actions might make them more sensitive to energies and beings. Through your work, they can deal with traumas and challenging emotions while fortifying their energy bodies, boundaries, and radiance. Listen closely, assess your clients, and offer them the tools, practices, and healing work to support them wherever they are. Do so in a way that doesn't wrap them up in extra stories about how sensitive or vulnerable they are or how they are harboring darkness or hosting an entity. There are ways to support people to be energetically robust and have better boundaries and self-care without scaring them.

16

SPEAKING IN TONGUES AND OTHER WEIRD STUFF

Self-love means embracing the weird parts.

During my awakening, a strange thing occurred. As I sat in meditation, overwhelming energy moved through my body. Peculiar sounds and words haltingly escaped my lips. Uncomfortable and confusing, streams of words moved through me. These came in languages I had never heard. I was aware of religious groups that spoke in tongues, but I had never seen it in real life or the media. Many call this speaking in light language, soul language, or light codes.

This was an integral part of opening my channel and speaking the words of another being, yet it was something I hid from others for a long time. It felt weird and, in a way, shameful. What did it mean? Was it real, or was I making it up? But the more I surrendered and allowed, the easier it came through me. The less I focused on what it meant, the more it had meaning. It flowed with power, taking form from the formless; this nonsensical nonsense wasn't that at all. It made perfect sense.

There are beings that speak these languages through me that I have come to recognize. Certain "words" and phrases have stuck with me from the beginning. These are prayers that I repeat over and over. They help create the trance that opens my channel. They call my helper beings and turn on my healing gifts. These phrases quickly and easily shift my consciousness. At a deeper level, it feels as though my soul can speak without the filter of this lifetime. At other times, there are streams of strange languages in tones and voices I have never heard before. This is usually when I tap into something connected to someone else, which happens in a healing or channeling session. I believe it also helps to shift the person's consciousness, to pull them out of mind space so they can receive on a subtler plane.

As these strange languages came through me, it was as though I understood what I was saying on a deep soul level but didn't have the precise translation into English. I struggled with this for years. I couldn't explain what it was or why it was. But the more I did it, especially in group healing sessions, the more I was allowed the translations. At first, they were halting and broken; over time, they flowed and were more accessible. Sometimes, when I deliver a message, it comes through in these languages because I can speak to the person on the soul level. To say it in English involves the rational mind, which strives to figure things out and take action. Some messages don't need to be processed by the mind. They are for the soul to know and feel.

Along with these languages come songs. I tune into someone's field and sing tones that shift their consciousness, open and move blockages, and heal. They are, of course, healing themselves. I tap into the needed frequency and bring it forward through sound. Some songs sound Native American, Japanese, European, or from a religious sect. These are for the person to receive. They are connected to their soul or guides, and they are their soul songs. We all have soul songs. These songs have been forgotten. When we remember them, we gain access to untapped energy and power. Some songs and languages come from the natural world. These are the songs of water, trees, and the Earth herself. To sing them is an honor and an honoring. They are powerful, sometimes sad and painful, sometimes joyful and sweet. They invoke the spirits of plants and animals, asking for their support and guidance.

Contained within these experiences are messages. I aim to get out of the way so they flow through. I accept that first, they might come through in these tongues, and then, as the energy integrates with my system, the translation will emerge naturally. I also accept that, at times, I will only get the translation in an energetic transmission afterward. This process is an ever-unfolding surrender into the present moment, relaxing the mental chatter and analysis to create the space for what is most needed.

The songs and speech that come through me have many uses and are involved in clearing, activating, encoding, and transmitting. They are a part of the more extensive journey of my personal practices and healing work.

Glossolalia

The phrase "speaking in tongues" troubles people. Many who attended Pentecostal or Charismatic Christian churches as children were traumatized to witness people shake, throw themselves to the ground, moan, and talk in gibberish while they drooled and sweated. People seem physically and psychically out of control in this state. This makes us highly uncomfortable, and we wish to control and explain it as quickly as possible. We might see it as a trick or the result of a hypnotic trance a religious leader puts people into, placing it into the realm of hoaxes. It is common practice for religious leaders to incorporate many trance-inducing techniques, which you can recognize if you know what to look for. The cadence and inflections they use and the incorporation of music and tones at key points shift consciousness. They combine this with working the energy of the collective along with other techniques.

Others see speaking in tongues as an authentic mystical experience. No matter what you think about seeing it in others, it can shake your whole foundation when it happens to you. After all, what seems crazier than spouting out a series of syllables and phrases that make no sense, sometimes in a shaking, writhing heap on the floor? But if this is part of your path, as it has been mine, learning to own, love, and use it in your work is invaluable.

Linguists have a beautiful word for speaking in tongues,

"Glossolalia." It is defined by the fluid vocalizing of speech-like syllables that lack any readily comprehended meaning, sometimes as part of religious practice. It is believed to be a divine language unknown to the speaker. It derives from the term glōssais lalō, a Greek phrase used in the New Testament meaning "speak in, with, or by tongues (other languages)." It has been chiefly studied and noted through witnessing various Christian religious groups from all over the world. They attribute it to the Holy Spirit, moving or speaking through a person. It has been observed in the Vodou tradition of Haiti and in the Hindu Gurus and Fakirs of India, and certain gnostic magical texts seem to be written in a description of this type of speech pattern.

Studies using MRI of people speaking in tongues have shown that the areas of the brain that translate thought to speech aren't lit up in the same way as when praying in a native tongue or using a mantra. The brain is in a deeply meditative space during the process. Further studies have shown that those who speak in tongues regularly report being happier and more satisfied with life.

Our logical brains are always trying to figure things out. If I tell someone something in English, they can mull it over, twist it about, and think on it until they destroy the true meaning or manipulate it into something else. It brings them into their analyzing brain and removes them from feeling and healing. When I speak to them on a soul level through this other way of communicating, they often tell me that they knew what I was saying on a deep level, but not one they can continue to analyze. It bypasses the part of the brain trying to figure everything out and instead opens up intuitive and soul-level aspects to receive in an entirely new way.

When "weird" things in spiritual work or healing sessions happen, your mind will judge. You will have doubts, insecurities, and possibly fear. You aren't alone. You're not crazy. This is quite common, and anything that starts to come through you isn't a one-off experience. It is easier on your body and other systems to allow these things to flow instead of holding them back with judgment and analysis. I encourage you to see if this is a part of your work and path. If strange sounds or phrases come through during one of the practices, go with it.

One of the keys to activating this is toning and singing that isn't focused on words. Stretch and open your mouth and jaw wide, roll your tongue, stretch it in every direction as far as possible, and allow your tones to be long and variable. Make sounds as you create random consonants to open the energy. Stretch and move your neck and release the need for your sounds to be beautiful or make sense. This is like creating art. You set up all the tools, get them ready, and hold space for something new and unknown to come through. Combine this with your invocation work, tune into a guide for support, and see what emerges. This practice can begin your journey of speaking out messages, healing sounds, or songs. Try not to judge yourself if it doesn't happen or feel natural. There are many gifts and many paths, and not everything will resonate.

Pain, Emotions, and Other Ugly Stuff as You Transmute Energies

Your work, like mine, might not always feel easy. We are in a time of great transmutation, requiring us to be present to darkness and intense emotions. Focus on your self-work to be as clear, grounded, and resourced as possible so that what you witness doesn't trigger repressed and stored emotions and energies.

As the magic people awaken and are called to release the energies of their repression, you might access images, memories, or experiences in sessions. You might see or feel a past life death or memory as if it is happening to you. This might be anchored to you, a client, or the collective. Many are called to work in the collective at this time, and as you transmute these energies for the group consciousness in your personal healing practices, you might access incredible pain. It can take a while to move through you. Your movement, breath, and sound practices are vital to maintaining your centered presence in these works.

I explored earlier how judgment and attachment to stories can hold you back. In your self-work or client sessions, you might experience memories, visions, or sensations. You can allow them to move through or focus on them intensely, giving them energy with your thoughts and words. Of course, it is valuable to inquire about what is to be learned from this information, but there can be a tendency to over-analyze and place value on what you experience. The more you let the images or awareness move through you without attachment, the better. If they stick, meaning there are repetitive thoughts or feelings about the experience, go back into yourself and your work, do your cleansing and purification practices, and ask for support to access and clear what might be connected to your personal story. Don't hold too tightly to what comes up in your sessions. You are giving it too much energy. It is moving through to be cleared. Allow that to happen. Too much focus on the memories, visions, or felt sensations can solidify identity around them or give them more energy to keep living inside the body or field of your client. You might want to discuss these things, so choose a mentor to help you process your experiences. Notice if you're telling stories to others about your experiences to feed excitement and sensationalism. Your work is sacred, and it is up to you to hold it as such.

When you go into channel space and bring through what is there, you can transmute lower-level energies through your system with the assistance of the light. I have channeled times, places, and environments for a long time, and when it first happened, it was intense and scary. Many people are waking up to do this work as we shift frequencies. If we can be fully surrendered, open, and call in all of our support, we can do this safely—which feels intense but moves massive energy. We can transmute energy in the environment and allow the light to work on us simultaneously. Again, I caution you to go slowly and take care of yourself. Don't attempt to transmute highly toxic areas unless you know exactly what you're doing, are extremely energetically sourced, and can take care of yourself afterward. Toxic regions of mass murder, war, or significant environmental damage are now being cleaned up by lightworkers. This work is best done in a collective with a powerful and capable leader and group.

In sessions, I access old instruments of torture and trauma that are related to the persecutions and subjugations of the magic and nature-based people. As I remove these, it helps people find their power and voice and access the wisdom of that lifetime. In that, I sometimes see and feel things like I am there, experiencing moments no one wants to observe. There is incredible pain, fear, and torment. I am a witness. I can't hold onto it, or it will harm me. I must do my own clearing work to not hold onto what I observed. I won't fully live my purpose if I am afraid to feel or go into these disturbing moments of pain. Ultimately, though I might describe the experience as painful (so you can relate to what I am sharing), it is heightened sensation, emotion, and energy, classified as pain because of our limited vocabulary.

You may encounter this type of work or the transmutation of energy of a place. This can feel overwhelming, but remember it isn't yours, and you don't have to hold it to be present and witness it enough to shift the energy. Use the same techniques you learned in The Healer's Process: grounding, sourcing, opening, cleansing, and purifying the area and yourself, and closing the container afterward.

17

CORD-CUTTING

Sometimes, the best medicine is to cut the cords that bind.

The energetic tendrils of our systems intertwine like vines through our bodies, hearts, and spirits. When we love someone deeply or sustain a long-term relationship (even if love isn't the reason we are connected), we are as energetically invested in them as they are in us. As if we share cells, we are much more interconnected than we would like to think.

You've felt this when a relationship ends. It feels like there is a hole in your heart or part of your body is missing. Even if you know the relationship doesn't work, you're in emotional, physical, and spiritual pain. They say time is the best medicine for healing all wounds, but that isn't always the case. Energy practices assist the process no matter what stage of healing.

Psychics and seers often witness cords embedded in people's bodies. Sometimes, these cords are draining energy. Cutting cords is an essential self-care practice. It should be done regularly to keep any client cords from embedding. It is imperative at the end of relationships. Times of transition are often when people seek out healers for support. They need help clearing energy from the former partner while witnessing emotions and assisting in life strategies. Cord cutting can be a beneficial part of healing work, not only when ending a romantic connection but also transitioning from any relationship.

A client was stuck in a repetitive breakup and re-engagement cycle. After our clearing work, she felt stable and unbothered by her former partner's overtures. She chose not to open any form of communication with him again, allowing the relationship to end with more ease. Many clients come for clearings at the end of relationships. It is common for people to feel deep yearning and longing, which binds them into toxic cycles. Cord cutting helps shift these painful and destructive dynamics.

Knowing a dynamic is unhealthy isn't always enough to create change. When the energetics are cleared, it is easier to distance from the repetitive thoughts and desires that often accompany deeply embedded cords. Cord cutting gives the opportunity to experience a different perspective and make self-preserving choices. Cord cutting can also be used to help people disengage from toxic work relationships and family members.

There are healthy and unhealthy cords, and these energetics can change over time. A mother corded to her child is beneficial as it creates a psychic and emotional bond that helps keep the child safe. During adolescence, there is a natural and often painful severing of this cord so the child can become independent and eventually find love and relationships. If this natural severing does not occur, it can create confusion. We have all heard of and seen movies portraying the grown man so connected to his mother that he can't sustain a romantic relationship.

You may fear that cord-cutting will disengage you from beneficial or loving relationships. This isn't the case. The energetics inspired by your intentions have an intelligence. Clearing cords, even with those you love, can support your inner clarity and discourage harmful dynamics.

People become corded to people but also places and things. You can see this in habituated patterns that are hard to break, addictions, and obsessions. Think about what it might look like if you could see all the energetic tendrils of your life. Some will be wispy and easy to break. Others will have more substance.

Creating Your Own Practice

There are many ways to cut cords. I offer suggestions, but this is your unique practice. Experiment and see what feels right. Do your foundational work of shaking, grounding, and sourcing so you can use that gathered energy to help remove and clear unhelpful cords. Intuitively feel into the fields and body, as you have learned earlier. Discover where you sense drains, cords, ropes, visions or thoughts of other people, or changes of density. Use your hands and the exhale breath, along with the intention to cut any cords that are not serving your highest. Work through your field, using cutting motions with your arms as you clear the cords. If you don't feel or sense much, you can still do the movement practice with your arms while focusing on your intention and breath. You will receive benefits and develop more intuitive awareness over time.

Be sure to refill the areas with light to purify. Don't worry that you might cut beneficial cords, such as to your partner. Clearing these cords, even with those we love, can help reset our center and clear any toxic energy collected from conflict in the relationship. You can then intentionally reconnect from a more empowered place. Work on this for yourself, and then bring this to your client sessions.

It is also helpful to do life assessments. People experience feeling drained or lacking energy and vitality and do not know why. Things become more apparent when they assess energy drains in their lives, which can include relationships but also social media, porn, and their work. With clients, this gives you a good idea of where to address energetically and how to coach them on life changes.

JOURNAL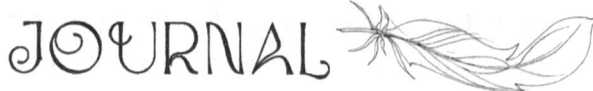

Feel into the cords in your life.

- Which are supportive and nurturing?

- Which are draining and holding you back?

- What energy and movement practices benefit cutting, clearing, and nurturing your field?

- What life changes are you willing to make?

[Practice 47: Cord Cutting]

[Practice 48: Cord Cutting in Sessions]

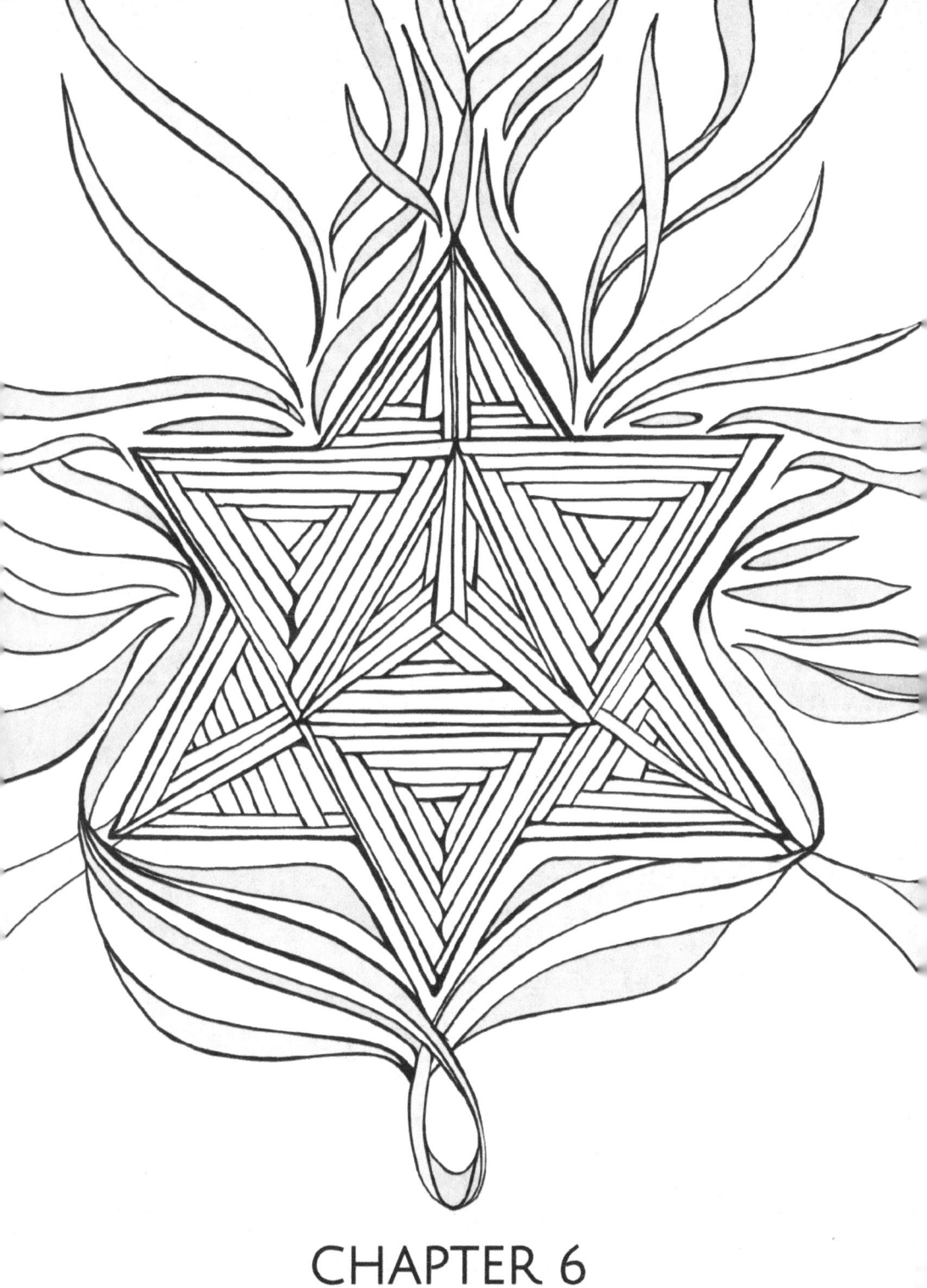

CHAPTER 6
INTEGRATION

CHAPTER 6

INTEGRATION

This is the shortest chapter designed to support the previous sections in calling you constantly back to deeper integration. You can't stay in constant expansion. Being in alignment with the natural flow of energy requires stillness and reflection. It also demands devoted actions and life changes. Awakening or magical experiences that aren't integrated into daily transformations of self don't have much value. It is easy to get distracted on this path by the mystical and sublime. It takes effort to discover how your new awareness or abilities make you a better human every day.

At the beginning of the book, I discussed how healing brings one back to wholeness. You have discovered many ways to do this through embodiment, energetic awareness, emotional intelligence, spiritual development, and healing inner parts. You have been calling yourself home and activating your beingness. The discovery of wholeness requires deepening integration cycles as you more fully embody and express the most aligned truth of your soul.

In this chapter, I will discuss how you can support your clients through their integration and further integrate your Healer's Process.

I invite you to sit with all you have learned and shifted as you allow your inner healer to emerge more fully from within you.

The topics in this chapter include:

- What to do after sessions.

- How to support your clients or yourself through a healing process.

- How to embrace yourself as a healer, mentor, and teacher.

- Bringing your work to the world.

1

AWARENESS AND RECEPTIVITY

It doesn't matter what mystical experiences
you've had if they don't inspire life changes.

Integration is the aspect of our work and lives we most often overlook. It took running The Healer's Process course several times before I said, "Hey! Why is there no integration module?!" Even after that, I left it out when reviewing the modules during the next retreat. We are all guilty of forgetting integration.

Our fast-moving consumer society places little value on rest and integration. I feel fortunate that, as a child, I wasn't involved in many extracurricular activities to the extent that so many children are today. I remember doing whatever I wanted to as a child after school or during the summer. Often, I was alone, not accomplishing much but having a lovely time. Now, it seems there is so much informed structure from when we are born till we die. We can see the effects of chronic exhaustion, overwhelm, self-medicating, and adrenal fatigue in our society. We go from one thing to the other as fast as we can. We judge rest harshly, and many are highly uncomfortable with it.

Most people also take this approach to healing. From the one seeking support, there is the thought, "I am going to go to someone, and they will do something to me, and then I will have the change that I want." From the practitioner, "Someone comes, I do stuff to or with them, they have the desired change."

Unfortunately, healing often doesn't work that way. Massive energetic shifts or ah-ha moments can occur in the office, retreat, or workshop. Everything seems cleared up and "fixed," yet the client slides back into illness, disease, or old patterns because they don't understand integration.

People go from workshop to training to retreat, one after the other. They are coached by several coaches, psychics, healers, and shamans in programs, medicine ceremonies, sound healings, and trips to sacred lands. They never stop. After all, when you're raised to believe that more is always better, you take that same approach to healing and transformation.

Have you been, or are you this person? Will you skim through this book, not do the exercises, and move on to the next text or course? Are you doing another training in a modality before you seriously practice and master the last one? You aren't bad for doing this. You're living out patterns enforced upon you at a young age.

JOURNAL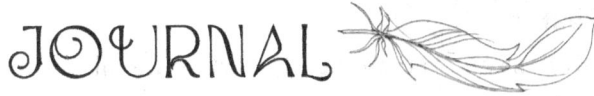

I encourage you to sit with (integrate) and ask tough questions about why you might do this.

- What was I taught about rest and inactivity as a child?

- Was I allowed to be bored?

- What is success to me?

- Do I believe I can succeed with what I have and who I am, or am I always one training away from being qualified enough to do my work?

- What do I get out of (or what I am avoiding by) overworking, overproducing, or overtraining?

Assimilation and Rest

Integration takes awareness and receptivity. It is when we allow our bodies and fields to assimilate the energetic and emotional changes initiated so they settle in and take root. It is also the process of doing homework, journaling, and making fundamental, concrete life changes that support the work at hand.

Integration also means rest. People are trained to be constantly busy, and rest isn't seen as valuable. Many experience health or personal crises because they refuse to rest and take care of themselves. The crisis is often the wake-up call not to get someone to "fix" them (as many think) but to make profound life changes in all areas.

Our lives and energy bodies are models for others. We can't expect our clients to do what we will not. This means instilling and sticking to daily practices that support who we want to be in the world.

Over the years, I have learned to pull back my energy and not give so much that it is a detriment. I allow more space for my clients and students to discover from themselves and their experiences, and I offer the integration time needed for the type of work I do. I pad more time in my programs and add integration-focused aspects to my work. So often, we want to give it all and create massive transformation in a way that isn't sustainable for our clients and their lives. At some point, I realized some of my desire to give was not coming from a place of personal fullness and solidity but from wanting to be seen as valuable and, in turn, to be loved. It's not a pretty realization to have. As facilitators and healers, we are constantly offered the opportunity to look at our shadow aspects and step more firmly into wholeness. Part of this might be pulling back in your work, providing less instruction, and focusing less intensely. This is your minimum effective dosage. There is no need to overdose someone on your power and energy. Analyze what amount you can give that will create change and opening without blowing out someone's system or sending them into a healing crisis.

JOURNAL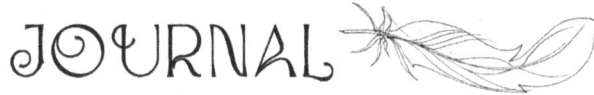

- When do I give too much in my work, and what have I noticed about that?

- What does my inner work look like right now?

- Am I honoring reflection, rest, and integration?

- What would less doing and more being look like?

- Do I feel I am in balance and flow? What could support that?

[Practice 49: Integration Practice]

2

AFTER A SESSION

Deep work requires robust support.

I 've talked about procedures after a session in Chapter 4. These include clearing yourself and your space and shutting down the work and your channel. I am now sharing what is supportive at the end of a client session. Of course, you will develop and create this as you build your practice, depending on how you see people and your work. The end of the session can make or break someone's experience. We often get so excited about "The Work" that we forget that this person has to get up, be in traffic, pick up their kids, and make dinner. A few moments of quiet integration at the end of the session can make a big difference.

Learn to track your client to feel how much they can process after the session. Give time to offer homework and recommendations. Don't give too much at once, or they won't do anything. You might want to send notes and homework afterward because people can be altered and integrating the energetics. Jumping into the logical brain can throw a wrench in the process. Assess their energy and where they are before analysis and homework. You might be closing a session where they have not gone into an altered state of consciousness so they can take in more instruction. Pay attention, track their energy and awareness, and use your intuition to give them what they need. Give one or two easy instructions at the end of the session, but only if it will be heard and assimilated.

Guide them with visualization or breathwork to bring them home fully in their body and conscious at the end of the session. They may have visited places they have not been since childhood. Perhaps they purged something old or upgraded their system. Bring them into awareness and help them integrate their experiences to reflect on what has happened and make realizations as needed. Make time for this! One of the reasons for the Healer's Process format is to track the session's needs and allow for what is coming up in every moment, knowing that certain aspects must be accomplished so you don't run over and leave things feeling unfinished or hanging. This gives the client a sense of safety and trust.

I often guide people to bring through information from aspects of themselves, their higher self, or guides. If I can, I will record or write down what came through. In these spaces, words melt away quickly, so if it feels valuable, find a way to hold onto it for them. Revisiting messages that came through them gives powerful anchors to your work together.

Always give your client time at the end of the session to integrate and rest. This can be hard as you typically have a time constraint. Remember that traditionally, when someone is ill or suffering, they might be with a healer for several hours or days, perhaps with multiple healers and supportive community members. You are doing one or two-hour sessions sandwiched between carpools and work schedules. Your clients may not know they need to rest after a session or take it easy that night. You have to explain what will be most supportive, and telling them beforehand when scheduling the session is the most beneficial so they can plan ahead.

I know to schedule more time with people when doing deep work with them. I don't schedule back-to-back sessions like many practitioners. I don't plan many people in one day. While conscious of time restrictions, I hold space for as long as it seems right.

Sync your breathing and ground their energy so they leave feeling supported. Again, this can happen quickly when you are trained in your grounding practice.

Ensure they have water to drink after the session and keep snacks like nuts and warm tea to help them ground and become present again. They may need to tell you what came up for them. You're the only person they may be able to talk to about these things, and you can't rush them out the door if they are in the middle of something big. Using The Healer's Process, you can cultivate the skill of adequately tracking your sessions to close and give space for integration. You will get better at this over time, but in these realms, the absolute gold can happen at the very end when someone has a realization about themselves and then shares that with someone they trust.

3

AFTER DEEP CLEARINGS AND EXTRACTIONS

Why yes, that was a nasty entity we extracted.

eep clearings, extractions, and removals of entities or implants leave an energetic, open wound that must be healed, nurtured, and loved. Just like a physical wound, areas of psychic surgery need aftercare. This essential self-care and integration should be included in practitioners' protocols. If you're called to do this work, educating your clients about their part in the healing process is vital. I have already discussed how many people give over the responsibility of their healing to a practitioner. Yet, self-care, inner work, and life changes are vital for long-term transformation. Knowing this, you must be prepared to guide them through the next best steps so they receive the most benefit.

Tell your client, "We have done some intense clearing work, so the next forty-eight to seventy-two hours are very important. Please pay attention to your surroundings and what you expose yourself to. Extra sleep, rest, and nurturing food are important. Take a break from the news and, if possible, social media entirely. Do your best to be around positive people and situations and avoid toxic people and environments. Take time to meditate, pray, be in nature, or focus on your breath each day."

"This is the primary area where we were working (tell them what areas of the body were being addressed). Keep this area covered and warm. Place your hands here and feel energy or light radiating into the area. Be gentle and kind to yourself. You may experience old emotions, fear, or uncomfortable sensations in your body as old patterns and energies are cleared from you further. Be aware that you might be more emotionally raw and sensitive right now. Be conscious of your interactions so you don't direct unhelpful outbursts on others. It is normal to feel like crying or yelling as old grief and anger move through you. Yoga, Qi Gong, gentle stretching, dance, walking, and breathwork will help move energy and emotions. Try to be present with your feelings and not shut them down, even if they are uncomfortable. You might benefit from journaling at this time."

After an extraction, I also suggest the person not only keep the area covered but, if possible, with something that feels protective or sacred. This might be a scarf from a holy site or a piece of jewelry with personal spiritual significance. It is helpful to keep a tall, glass pillar candle lit near the bed and to burn incense or resins, which will help to cleanse and purify the home. I will also offer people prayers and statements of sovereignty, such as the ones you have learned in this book or from texts that resonate with their spiritual beliefs. I also encourage baths with Epsom salt, essential oils, and herbs. Simple herbs they might already have or can easily purchase are beneficial, such as rosemary, thyme, roses, and sage.

People are creatures of habit. They don't think about what they do, where they go, or what they consume through food, drink, or visually. It is good to remind them that prayer, gratitude, love, and laughter will help them heal, while negative, fear-based interactions and media will have the opposite effect. This is an excellent time to avoid bad habits and begin new, simple ones that are not hard on the body. When someone hears this instruction, they might think you are telling them to take up an extreme diet or work out daily because this is the social conditioning of replacing habits. Small changes such as walking daily and soaking in the tub will best serve them. You can use information from your assessment process and conversations to help them discover what will work best for them.

After sessions, people are more open. Their field is repairing and regenerating. These can be vulnerable moments. There is no need to scare your client, but use reminders that empower and assist.

Often, clients want to go to a practitioner to get an energy clearing but don't know to follow up on the deeper work required. People get attachments and other challenging issues because they are vulnerable. They have opened themselves up in some way. This might have been during a traumatic situation in the past, but it might indicate a more long-term break in the field, resulting from co-dependence, faulty boundaries, energy leaks, thought forms and beliefs, addictions, and childhood wounds. These issues can be dealt with in subsequent sessions to complete the healing, but your client must be made aware of these interdependent issues. This will help shore up the system so it isn't vulnerable in the future, requiring the same clearings repeatedly. As healers, we help people to change their consciousness, habits, beliefs, and underlying reasons for the physical, energetic, spiritual, and emotional issues they are experiencing.

People tend to see cords, attachments, entities, or the like as issues outside of themselves that a practitioner is "removing," and that is the end of it. On the contrary, these powerful teaching moments allow people to learn, heal, and grow. You are in charge of helping your client understand the larger picture. If they are ill or struggling, things must change beyond clearing their field or releasing their muscles. For complete integration of your work, it's important to acknowledge the deeper aspects of forgiveness, emotional release, nervous system repair, and shifting life patterns.

It is beneficial to share some of the cleansing and purification practices you have been learning with your clients. This is especially important for those who have had significant attachments, as they need to cleanse and purify their homes. This is why it's important to do your personal practices where you discover what is most supportive and share from a place of mastery and experience.

4

SUPPORTING YOUR CLIENTS

Integrating supportive practices can be
as healing as the session itself.

People are waking up at lightning speed, and we are often integral catalysts to these awakenings. Authentic, powerful work produces authentic, powerful experiences. These include sudden and intense shamanic and psychic awakenings, kundalini and energetic activations, and emotional catharsis.

Even great healers can make the mistake of opening a client too quickly, leaving them lost, confused, scared, and unable to manage their experience. Those who have always had psychic and intuitive gifts or did not have an intense awakening can sometimes not know what to do with these clients. Many clients have come to me because they experienced an opening with another practitioner, and the practitioner didn't know what to do with the client's sudden psychic abilities, sensitivities, or memories surfacing. Often, the client is left feeling abandoned when the practitioner doesn't know what to do or who to refer them to next.

It is often necessary to give context to people about what they are experiencing, even if it seems simple to you. We often get so used to the magical, feeling-based life that we forget this might be new to others, even ones who seem to have been on a spiritual or personal development path for a while. If you don't want to explain what is happening in someone's system as they awaken and heal, find someone to refer them to for learning supportive practices. The practices in this book are not only for you but for you to share with your clients, especially those struggling with an intense awakening.

It's dangerous to leave someone overwhelmed with visions and hearing things over which they have no control because you haven't taught them anything about navigating a psychic or shamanic awakening. This might not be your specialty. As I have said before, having other practitioners you can refer to is crucial when people need more support.

Often, people need more than anything to be told they are okay, their experiences are normal, and they are not in danger. They want to know you understand, and they have at least one safe person to talk to about what is happening.

People might not feel better right away. They may be shifting and processing a lot of shadow frequency or ancestral wounding. Shamanic awakenings are often accompanied by frightening and dark imagery, overwhelming visions, or long, confusing experiences with spirits. Through the process, people can experience shamanic sickness or awakening flu, which doesn't clear for a while. This could feel like they are sick with a strange illness and have symptoms such as fever, sweats, nausea, ringing in the ears, exhaustion, or a host of bizarre flu-like symptoms that don't respond to treatment. Initiations and shifts in vibration can be unpredictable. Many people are unaware that this is a thing or that they might be the kind of person who could have this experience. Many have to deal with shadow aspects of the archetypal energies they are awakening, as described in the I AM chapter. Understanding the archetypes will help you give your clients context for their experiences.

People are often nudged into dark nights of the soul in our care and need support in understanding the process. It doesn't feel good. It is the dying of all that was before. A new self will emerge, but it might take a while. They need to understand that you will shepherd them. So often, people will stop going to practitioners or feel they can't "be healed" because they are having a hard time. This is precisely when they need a supportive mentor to help them. Don't be afraid to follow up with your people and ask how they are doing. They might be struggling but afraid to reach out. Cheer on their victories but also the dark and uncomfortable parts. They are learning a new way of approaching and interacting with themselves. This approach integrates and accepts all aspects as they learn how to feel even the painful parts.

Your clients must understand that some parts are easy and shift quickly; some aspects require devotion and dedication. Internal blocks will come up. The more you prepare people for this, the more likely they will recognize it when it happens and ask for support. Practices and homework help them access their own inner power and healing potential. Trust yourself enough to offer practices and give homework. I have met practitioners who avoid doing this as they are not confident in their personal practice or don't want to impose it on their clients. Do your own work to the extent that you become confident in your integration offerings.

5

MENTOR AND TEACHER

A healer is never just a healer.

A s a healer, you are called into service, encompassing many different roles. You support people through illness and crisis, help them understand themselves and the world, and offer the tools they need to thrive. You might want to "do some things" to someone and send them on their way, but as I have said before, people must actively engage in their healing process. It's crucial to empower people to recognize their ability to heal themselves by adopting new ways of thinking and exploring their inner truths through consistent practice and introspection.

As you master yourself, you will discover that you have emerging gifts called into expression. You might see your role in your practice expand to encompass more than you previously considered. Perhaps you initially focused on specific issues, but as you gain a more holistic perspective, you see that people require support in numerous areas of their lives. This is exciting because it inspires you to grow and expand your toolbox. However, pushing the edge of who you have thought yourself to be can be intimidating as you take on a new role in someone's life. You become aware of your increased impact on others and your work's responsibility. You have the power to inspire and motivate positive change, acting as a catalyst for others to embrace their authentic selves and express their truth.

You may find yourself assuming the role of a teacher and mentor, requiring you to shift your focus and embrace new parts of yourself. Teaching and sharing bring confidence and mastery. The practices and concepts outlined in this book and those learned in other trainings should not be kept to yourself. Instead, they should be shared with the world to benefit others. You may even encourage your people to share what you have brought into their lives. In this way, you can have a more significant impact on the planet as we collectively shepherd the awakening we are all eager to see.

As a guide on the path, it is important to acknowledge that you may not always have the perfect answer. Be honest about your limitations and meet people where you are. There is no need to inflate yourself or put on a mask of perfection. Your journey has provided you with valuable wisdom, which is to be shared.

You may see that some of the work you are called to do is held within the container of being a parent or guide for children. These young ones have heightened sensitivity and are attuned to their surroundings. They possess an intuitive and energetic understanding that we, as adults, have long forgotten. Right now, children are more "remembered" than ever before. Many are coming in at a level of consciousness that we can't comprehend. Yet, there is a lack of instruction regarding their energetic or emotional bodies and the spiritual realms. They need easy ways to do this work early on so they are not damaged and need to seek this help as adults. They need support to master their gifts and abilities. If you are a parent, share playfully some of the teachings you have learned. Shaking, tapping the body, breathing big, holding the breath, and sending it out with a loud sound are all fun. Simple prayers, clearing practices, and using the imagination to focus on colored light assist difficult sleepers and little ones seeing things "that aren't there."

I believe it is possible for healers to lead from the middle, to guide as we walk side by side with our people. We are all walking each other home. Lean into the awareness that we are all healers. Every person you work with will offer you a way to grow. Each person is a valuable contributor to the overarching goal of transformation. We must respect and honor each individual's unique path, even if it is messy or involves significant pain and trauma. Ultimately, each journey adds value to our unfolding mission.

As you learn how to lead from this new dynamic, you allow yourself and others to shine.

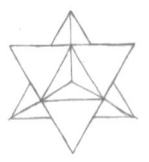

THE WELL

You are the owner of a well.

*You have been digging this well for years. You put in hard labor.
You studied with great well masters so that it is strong and deep.*

*The land is dry and barren. Water is scarce. A woman with no water
travels through the heat to your land, seeking that which will sustain
her life. You share the water because it is the only thing you can do.
You reach deep into the well and pull forth the life-nourishing liquid.*

The woman thanks you and goes away.

*You worry if the water might make her sick. Maybe you didn't
pull from deep enough or filter out enough sediment.*

You worry that she will tell others.

*You worry that you might not have enough in your
well if many people know you have this gift.*

*You worry that others will look at you differently if
you are a well owner. You might feel separate.*

*Slowly, they appear. At first, one or two at a time. Soon,
families. They set up camps to cook and sleep because yours is
the closest water for many miles. A community develops.*

At this point, you have a decision to make.

Do you close the well to save the precious juice
for yourself? Do you send the thirsty people away
knowing they might not find water elsewhere?

Do you deny owning the well so you are not
responsible for all these people?

Do you pretend you don't have this water because you don't
want to be celebrated? After all, this might inflate your ego.

Who are you to own a well?

Who are you to supply life to those thirsting?

Are you willing to take on this responsibility?
The gift handed by the great Mother?

Will you reach deep inside to bring forth life for others?

The land is parched. The people thirst.

You own the well. Own it well.

6

AVOIDING DOGMATISM

Many spiritual paths enforce rigidity over flexibility.

A
s you walk your path of healing and spiritual evolution, you will encounter many teachers and teachings. You will learn various modalities and processes. Some will resonate, and others will not. In my studies, I have observed that there can be a lot of limitations and restrictions. Often in a workshop or training, you may hear, "Never do this," "Never talk about that," "No, that doesn't happen with clients," or "No, you can't do that until you have completed this particular training at the end of the three-year program." This is often in response to people naturally having things arise that they aren't "supposed" to do yet. This might be having past life visions while working, sensing the spirits of deceased loved ones, or matter of factly, removing dark and disturbing energies from someone's body.

There is a lot of "no" energetics out there. In a way, this makes sense. Someone has studied a great deal, formulated a process, and hopefully rigorously tested it with many people and practitioners, and this is their system. They want it taught and done a certain way to be as effective and safe as possible. Additionally, they are usually vested in maintaining ownership and control over their modality or brand. Teachings of lineages must be respected so they are not lost to our over-consumptive tendencies to make everything our own.

Some advanced energy practices without instruction or preparation can cause issues in the energy system or a breakdown, so they must be done with specific considerations. I have repeatedly told you not to put yourself or others at risk by avoiding your inner work and personal practices and developing your skillset. What I am talking about here is the dogmatic way that many modalities are taught. Some are taught with so many rules and restrictions that the love and excitement for the work are squeezed out. I've learned practices I loved, but then I was told it was the only way to get a result or move forward. I've been instructed not to mix this water practice with that fire practice, not to do a Yoga practice with a particular meditation practice, not to wear crystals while doing this treatment, not to do anything intuitive in an energy healing modality, not to see visions, to stick rigidly to a protocol, and not mix this healing practice with any other healing practice.

It can leave people feeling that if they aren't performing a specific set of practices correctly, they are inadequate, flawed, and not safe, effective, or powerful in their healing work or life. This reminds me of the rigid and often oppressive principles that run and ruin many religions.

People love dogma. There appears to be a deep-seated longing to be told what to do. We have an intense desire to execute tasks flawlessly and adhere to a prescribed set of actions that will lead us to salvation, mastery, enlightenment, or any other desired outcome.

I've never been fond of "no" and "never." The concept of only one path to follow is unsettling to me. How could that be? I've observed that those with a higher level of enlightenment tend to be less dogmatic. They appear to maintain an elevated consciousness that all paths lead to the same destination as long as they are approached with an open heart and mind, the right intentions, and create beneficial relationships with self, others, and the world. This orientation might serve you if you train in modalities that seek to restrict and confine your magic into a box built by another. Remember your true self, the one you have been exploring here, even in the midst of another's power.

It is beneficial to commit to a path and see it through to its fullest to gain valuable knowledge, insight, and ability. I encourage you to study and take in as much as possible of a lineage or teacher.

But, there are many paths and so much inner wisdom and personal connection to Source to explore. Don't limit yourself by becoming so enamored of a teacher that you lose your intrinsic knowledge. Remain watchful and take everything with a grain of salt. Don't let anyone absorb your purpose by diminishing your inner light or trust in yourself.

Always notice when your practice feels stale, when you are on autopilot, when you aren't inspired, and in those moments, go more deeply into yourself and learn something new and entirely different to stretch your concepts of how things are done. Open your system to receive the flow of information, wisdom, and processes from your guides, your lineage of truth. Follow the synchronistic trail to your own way of working.

EPILOGUE

TRUST YOURSELF

Throughout these pages, I have shared my thoughts with you, hoping to provide guidance and advice. At times, I am sure I've seemed certain, righteous, and right, but my words are not the only truth. I am a person, the same as you. There will be differing opinions from others you study with. I hope that you find what works best for you.

The most important thing on this journey is to express yourself. Maybe you don't know what that looks like right now. Maybe you've seen glimpses of it. Perhaps you're quite connected to your truth. There is more. There is more truth inside you waiting to be spoken, sung, danced, and shared. You are needed in this world — you, the unique expression of you. You know more than you give yourself credit for.

Once you accept that you are an expression of the Divine, you can live as such. It isn't always easy. Often, there are dark times on the journey of becoming whole and expressed. All of your shadows will rise to the surface. Allow yourself to play with them. It is the only way.

The more you discover who you are, the more connected you are in your relationships and life. The more you express your truth, the more it bubbles up to the surface.

One of the greatest gifts is trusting yourself.

You are wise. You are strong. You can do this. Being yourself is the most profound contribution you can give to this world.

I am cheering you on.

SPECIAL BOOK BONUS RESOURCES

Gain access to free special resources and education associated with
The Healer's Process:

https://katherinebird.com/the-healers-process-bonus/